Living with
Type 2
Diabetes

other books by Gloria Loring

The Days of Our Lives *Celebrity Cookbook*
Kids, Food, and Diabetes
Parenting a Child with Diabetes

other books by Dr. Timothy Gray

Backworks: The Illustrated Guide to How Your Back Works and What to Do When It Doesn't
Osteoporosis: The Silent Stalker

Living with Type 2 Diabetes

MOVING PAST THE FEAR

Gloria Loring
+
Dr. Timothy Gray, D.O.

PRESS™
Milwaukie

Book design by Heidi Fainza
Cover design by Lia Ribacchi & Heidi Fainza
Cover photograph by Bader Howar
Illustrations by José Marzan Jr.

M Press
10956 SE Main Street
Milwaukie, OR 97222

mpressbooks.com

Library of Congress Cataloguing-in-Publication Data available upon request.

ISBN-10 1-59582-016-7
ISBN-13: 978-1-59582-016-7
First M Press Edition: April 2006
10 9 8 7 6 5 4 3 2 1

Printed in U.S.A.
Distributed by Publishers Group West

TABLE of CONTENTS

acknowledgments

Thank you to Thorn and Ursula Bacon for shepherding this book to its completion; to Dr. Tim Gray for his dedication and enthusiasm; to Barbara Toohey and June Biermann for their inspiration; and to Dr. Irl Hirsch for his invaluable support. I appreciate the input I have been given from knowledgeable and compassionate health care professionals such as Kathy Lowe BSN, RN, CDE; Aulikki Brandt, former director of Bristol's Tennessee's Diabetes Treatment Center, and Debbie McClellan, RD, LDN, CDE. I send my love and appreciation to Deborah for all her help, proofreading, and encouragement. Most of all, to Brennan—dear one, I see and hear how difficult these years have been, and I pray you are delivered safely from this challenge someday soon.

introduction

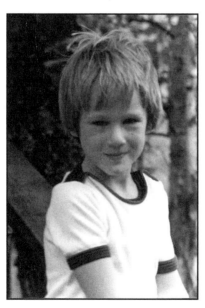

There was a time when I knew nothing about diabetes. That was before my son, Brennan, got it.

I remember that night. I watched as Brennan drank three glasses of water in quick succession. I asked his aunt, a nurse, what could cause a child to drink that much water. She told me it could be diabetes. My mind stopped. There was too much fear for it to hold. The fear continued through the education process at Children's Hospital Los Angeles. It almost wrestled me to the floor when the doctor told me that 50% of those with diabetes die within twenty-five years of diagnosis. When we took Brennan home, it whispered, "What if you do something wrong? What if you give him too much insulin or not enough food?" It still sings its song in me, at times. Times when I think of how long it's been, how long Brennan's body has endured its daily struggle for balance. Time when I hear that diabetes has taken a leg or a kidney or someone's eyesight. I refuse to listen to its rumblings. I turn my head and go back to what is true today: My son has lived with the d-word for almost twenty-seven years and he's doing fine. He's engaged to a beautiful, smart young woman and they are planning a wedding.

In the early days and weeks after his diagnosis, I learned to move past the fear that wanted to immobilize me. Even now, when it jumps into my heart, I'm able to put it aside. Fear doesn't have a firm foothold in my life because, from the beginning, I've had the support I've needed. I've been in contact with people who understand the challenges of diabetes. They've given me the information I needed. They told me of the dangers, but they also filled me with hope. Dr. Tim and I wrote this book to give you that kind of support. You can live successfully with Type 2 diabetes. You may even be able to become symptom-free. If you meet the challenges diabetes presents to you, you may find you're not quite the same person you used to be. That's not necessarily a bad thing.

When my son was first diagnosed, I was the girl least likely to stand up for anything. I would have said, "Who, me?" I was a singer and wasn't afraid to get up on a stage, but offstage I was not very confident. I'd been raised under the roof of my grandmother's mantra, "What will the neighbors think?" If you're always worried how your actions look to others, you're not likely to try anything too challenging.

That changed when my son asked me, "When will my shots be over?" How was I going to tell my four-year-old that the injections would last his whole life? I told him, "I don't know, but I'm working on it." I joined the Juvenile Diabetes Research Foundation and embraced their mission to find a cure for diabetes. I did things I'd never done before: I raised money for research, wrote and published books, and formed a record company. My confidence deepened and my people skills grew, all because Brennan got diabetes. Christian mystic Pierre Teilhard de Chardin said, "Not everything is immediately good . . . but everything is capable of becoming good." I agree.

So much has changed since Brennan was diagnosed. *This is the best time in the history of humanity to have diabetes*, because the medical community knows more about how to care for diabetes than ever before. Each year brings an increase in research dollars, improved treatments, and more effective medications. At the same time, diabetes is now considered an epidemic. A recent estimate put the number of people with Type 2 diabetes at 120 million worldwide. The prediction is that by the year 2010, this figure will reach 200 million and a larger percentage is younger than ever before. There has been a significant increase of Type 2 diabetes in children and younger adults: Of the 15 to 20 million with Type 2 diabetes in America, at least half were born between 1946 and 1964. One out of every three people born in the year 2000 will develop diabetes.

There are two obvious reasons for the alarming rise in Type 2 diabetes: poor diet and lack of exercise. More and more of us are eating in restaurants and grabbing fast food to go with our fast-paced lifestyle. Too many of us have settled into sedentary ways. Yet study after study has shown that by changing what we eat and adding appropriate exercise and medication, many people with Type 2 diabetes can bring their blood sugar levels very close to normal.

In my high school driver's education class, we were required to watch a movie about automobile safety produced by Ford Motor Company. (Of course, the cars that were driven safely were Fords and the cars that got into accidents were Chevys.) At the end of the film, they showed actual traffic accidents with bodies strewn on the highway. We got the message: "This can happen if you are not careful."

Most of this book is focused on the "Ford Motor Company" news about diabetes, but Dr. Tim and I also want you to know about the "traffic accident" news. I've heard too many people with diabetes complications say, "Nobody ever told me this could happen. If I'd known, I would have taken better care of myself." Your day-to-day care is in your hands. If you don't adequately control your blood sugar, diabetes will hurt you. Dr. Tim and I don't want that to happen—to you or to anyone.

This book is divided into twelve chapters. Chapter one, "Expect a Miracle," tells the story of what happened to me after Brennan was diagnosed. Chapter two, "A Short Course on Diabetes," describes what diabetes is and the role obesity plays in Type 2. Chapter three, "Yeah, Team!" guides you in assessing the health care professionals who will be educating and treating you. It provides goals for your doctor visits and physical examinations, and explains why each aspect is important. Chapter four, "What a Difference a Day Makes," presents the elements of daily diabetes management, the "how to" of blood sugar tests, oral medications, and a little primer on the psychological process of living with diabetes.

The complexities of insulin therapy are addressed in chapter five, "Everything is Upside Down." Chapter six is about "Food, Glorious Food" and how to make healthy choices. "Tote That Barge, Lift That Bale," chapter seven, discusses the whys and hows of exercise. Chapter eight, "Teach the Children Well" is for parents of children with diabetes and chapter nine, "Valley Low, Mountain High," ponders the fine points of blood sugar control, especially during sick days or travel.

Chapter ten, "Stress: The Tiger You Don't Want in Your Tank" offers strategies for reducing stressful responses. Diabetes' dark side—complications— and how to avoid them forms chapter eleven, "Dangers and Dragons." Chapter twelve, "We All Need a Hero," introduces you to people who have made the best of diabetes. There's an addendum of questions that Dr. Tim is most frequently asked, along with his answers, and a Resources for Readers section.

It is my voice coupled with Dr. Tim's expertise that you hear throughout this book. He has been in practice for thirty-five years and has treated hundreds of diabetic patients in his Oregon practice. Because of his extensive knowledge of diabetes, he developed a highly recommended Type 2 treatment protocol for family practice physicians. In addition, diabetes is a part of his family's heritage and he has had to work to keep his own blood sugar levels in good control.

We hope you'll use this book frequently during your first year of diagnosis and refer to it any time you are uncertain. As time goes by, perhaps you will become enough of an expert to consider writing your own book.

Gloria Loring
February, 2006

a family physician
learns about diabetes

In 1996 I confronted the problem that is typical of every family care physician: I didn't feel I was adequately helping people who came to me for answers about diabetes. In an office visit of fifteen to twenty minutes, I could not possibly cover all of the medical issues of Type 2 diabetes: blood pressure, foot care, eye exams, inspecting a patient's log book, and discussing exercise and blood sugar testing. Other physicians I talked to were as overwhelmed as I.

As a reminder of what I needed to cover, I made a 4 x 6 inch card listing crucial diabetes topics, sealed it in plastic, and carried it in my white coat pocket. The card helped, but often after the patient left my office, I would discover I had missed something.

I attended a program put on by the famed Joslin Diabetes Center to learn more about diabetes. I discovered that primary care doctors like myself treat ninety percent of patients with diabetes, often without a methodical program. When a patient with diabetes comes into the office these physicians are concerned they may omit some needed diagnostic tests or treatments. I decided the only way I could be fair and professional with my patients was to change my practice focus. I had done that before.

Several years ago, I had a disk injury while lifting weights. I was doing a 390 pound squat when I lost my balance and fought the barbell to the floor. I had a disk injury in my back and I developed a "foot drop." My foot would "catch" on the carpet when I walked. I left my position at a primary care clinic to work in a spine rehabilitation clinic to learn how to recover from my injury. I did recover and used the principles I learned to write a book, *Backworks—The Illustrated Guide to How Your Back Works and What to Do When It Doesn't*. It became a book-of-the-month club selection for *Prevention* magazine and Doubleday Health Book Club.

About the same time, I had an insurance physical and discovered that my blood sugar was elevated. My father and several relatives had diabetes, and some of them had complications that resulted in amputations. I knew I had to take that early warning seriously. I became "The Alien," as my daughter calls me. I bicycle ten miles a day. Five headlights illuminate my path and five flashing taillights on my bike, helmet, and backpack increase visibility from behind. I understand what it takes to control blood sugar levels. I also understand the challenge of caring for patients who have diabetes. I am one of the more than 125,000 primary care physicians across the country that are responsible for providing diabetes care with limited time and resources.

Then I attended a medical program that suggested that each practitioner decide how medicine should be practiced five or ten years in the future and start practicing that way now. As a result, we developed the position of "Chronic Care Coordinator." The coordinator is responsible for diabetes, congestive heart failure, asthma, and hypertension. She reviews each patient's chart the day before the appointment and places a summary of the problems that need to be addressed on the front page of the chart. This simple system has saved us hours of time leafing through charts looking for test results and chart notes.

Another source of help came from OMPRO, the Oregon Medical Professional Review Organization. It has developed a program for treating chronic medical problems. In cooperation with OMPRO, we are completing "The Diabetes Collaborative" with six other medical teams from Oregon. Our next step is to spread the information we have developed into treatment protocols for physicians in our community. It will give them better methods of treating diabetes and other chronic illnesses. Our diabetes program today is a true delight. With the use of our e-brain, the electronic medical record program, we can stay focused and address underlying problems, often before they become symptoms. We've also made arrangements with a fitness center and their trainers to work with our patients with diabetes and their partners at no charge.

I think we are starting to be effective. A patient of mine who is a former Denver Broncos football player recently complained, "I'm going to find a new doctor. I'm tired of all the reminders for physicals, lab tests, flu shots, and cardiac treadmills. I'm going to find a doctor who doesn't care so much."

I'm pleased to share the knowledge I've gained with you. I hope it helps you and your doctor provide great diabetes care for someone very important—you.

Dr. Tim Gray

. . . it's okay to expect
a miracle, even in
the face of seemingly
insurmountable odds.

chapter one

expect a miracle

It was July 1979. We were on a family vacation in Canada and my four-year-old son, Brennan, was exhibiting some unusual behaviors. His great-grandfather noticed that Brennan was drinking a lot of liquids and mentioned it to me.

"Well, it's summer, we're traveling, and it's hot," I reasoned.

Then Brennan started wetting the bed. He'd never done that before. I pieced together some reasons, "He's off his sleep schedule and he's drinking so much liquid because he's hot." He was also very fussy and cranky, not his usual sweet self. I noticed that the size six shorts that had fit him perfectly a month ago were now sliding down his hips. I watched him playing with his cousins. His face looked thinner than usual. Out of curiosity, I weighed him on the scale in his grandmother's bathroom. At the doctor's office six weeks earlier, Brennan had weighed fifty-one pounds. Now the scale read forty-six pounds. He'd lost five pounds? I didn't know what to make of it.

At one point during our travels, I turned to look at Brennan sitting behind me in the car. He was staring straight ahead as if mesmerized. His face was dry and flushed deep pink. His eyes were glassy. He had no fever, no outward signs of illness, but it was obvious something wasn't right. His father and I agreed we'd take him to the pediatrician when we got home in a few days.

That night, at our family reunion, Brennan shared a room connected to ours with his older cousin, Boyd. As I tucked him in, he asked for a glass of water. He drank it quickly. "More, Mommy." He drank a second glassful, then, to my amazement, a third. Boyd's mother was in the room and knowing that she was a nurse, I asked her, "What on earth could cause a child to drink that much water?"

Her answer was, "There's only one thing I can think of—diabetes."

There was a name for what was happening to Brennan. I had heard of diabetes, but knew nothing about it. We called Brennan's doctor and told him what we'd observed. He suggested we collect Brennan's first urine in the morning and get some test strips to see if he was spilling sugar. We lay in bed holding hands all night long, listening for Brennan. At six A.M. we heard him get up to go to the bathroom. We followed immediately and asked him to pee into the bathroom water glass. He was still too sleepy to question why. We dipped the test strip in. Dark blue. Sugar in the urine. Diabetes.

That first year after Brennan's diagnosis was very busy. We did some research and found the Juvenile Diabetes Research Foundation (JDRF), formed by parents of children with diabetes who were committed to finding a cure. We joined. While I struggled with Brennan's daily care, Alan created a fundraising project: a specialty record and video featuring hockey players. He told me creating the record was his way of working out his sadness over Brennan's diabetes.

His example sparked a little competitive spirit in me. If he could do it, so could I! Raising money for research would help to find the answer to Brennan's question, "When will my shots be over?" Since I didn't have any immediate ideas of how I was going to help JDRF, I decided to watch for a possibility.

Ten months after Brennan's diagnosis, I auditioned for the role of "Liz Chandler" on the daytime drama *Days of Our Lives*. I did well enough to be called back to read for the producers, and then screen-tested with three other actresses. I was hired.

My boys, Brennan, born in 1974 and Robin, born in 1977, had traveled with me for singing engagements since they were babies. I didn't want to give up singing and performing, but I also didn't want to be away from my children. Now it was May of 1980, just months before Brennan was to enter kindergarten and I got my first steady job, in Los Angeles, where I lived. No more travel. No more getting off of airplanes with two toddlers in tow, my clothes decorated with smashed banana. In addition to keeping me close to my children, *Days* provided another benefit. Being on a popular television show would provide me with a constituency from which to raise money for diabetes research.

In the first weeks after Brennan's diagnosis, he tolerated his daily insulin injections. As the months marched on, each morning's shot became a battle of wills. The urgency to inject lifesaving insulin was matched by Brennan's resistance. Some mornings dawned on a screaming and sobbing child restrained by one parent as the other plunged a needle into his small thigh. Those mornings, I understood what hell must be like.

How I could help him? How could I answer his question, "When will my shots be over?" The "how" revealed itself in the makeup room at *Days*, accompanied by the hum of hair dryers and rustling script pages. Each day, as faces were raised to individual heights of perfection, I listened as actors around me traded recipes. A few years before, I had been asked to contribute a recipe for a celebrity cookbook. Now an idea formed: I would assemble a *Days* cookbook to raise money for diabetes research!

I asked some questions and discovered that *Days* attracted more than ten million viewers a day, yet the show's owners had never created any major souvenir items for the fans. There were a few puzzles and coffee mugs, but nothing that featured a personal glimpse of the actors. A Dallas friend, John Hamilton, had once mentioned to me that there are ways to sell a book without "selling" it. That phrase had stuck in my mind and I called John for an explanation. He outlined an approach of offering a book as a "premium," an item given free with a purchase or given in exchange for a donation.

The Days of Our Lives Celebrity Cookbook was born. I formulated a plan to gather a picture, recipe, and personal autograph from each of the actors. Then I had to convince someone to underwrite the project and figure out the details of publishing and distributing it as a giveaway in exchange for a donation to JDRF.

In order to create and publish the cookbook, I had to develop a new sense of myself. If Brennan's diabetes had been something that might develop in the future, I might have been able to put off doing something, but I couldn't avoid facing what diabetes brought to Brennan's life each day. We'd been told that diabetes could shorten his life span by twenty-five years. There were insulin injections and blood tests. We worked to balance his food intake with the insulin dosage, trying to keep his blood sugar in the normal range. It was not an easy task to constantly monitor a small active, growing boy. Each day was a struggle.

My fear fueled my resolve. I would do whatever was needed to help my son. By creating the cookbook, I could trade my feeling of helplessness for activism. I assembled the recipes, autographs, and photos. Staff members at *Architectural Digest* recruited by a JDRF volunteer designed the graphics and typesetting, and got us a special discount on the paper costs through their supplier. Their printing company was lined up, ready to go. One small detail was missing: money. My presentations to corporations and private businesses for financial support had been politely rejected.

Getting everything ready to go to print took eight months and people at the studio kept asking me how the cookbook was coming along.

I'd smile and say, "Fine."

Not really. I was running out of ideas for how to raise $40,000 to print 50,000 cookbooks. I'd been told that what I was trying to do was not possible without the help of an influential publishing company. I was getting discouraged. I didn't realize there were some influences at work I hadn't counted on.

It was 6 A.M. on a Friday at NBC Studios; I put my carry bag on the chair in my dressing room. I took out my script and other essential items. Makeup, shoes.

I was "first up" that day. My scenes were being taped first, because I had to catch a plane to Houston to participate in the Jack Benny Memorial Tennis Classic to benefit JDRF. I finished my scenes and ran to the dressing room. I packed my bag and lifted it from the chair. On the seat of the chair was a card that read, Expect a Miracle. I picked it up and wondered out loud, "Where'd this come from? It wasn't here this morning."

I was about to throw the card in the trash when a little voice inside said, "Don't throw away a card that says Expect a Miracle!"

This was my first remembrance of an inner voice speaking to me. It didn't feel like my mind was thinking a thought. This felt like somebody was in my head, speaking with a tone of authority I didn't often have. I looked at the card and instead of tossing it in the trash can, I put it in my carry bag. I headed for the airport and Houston.

The next evening, after a day of round-robin tennis, I sang two songs as part of the evening's celebrity show. As I came down from the stage, a man who looked familiar was waiting for me.

"Gloria, it's Ben Rogers. Do you remember me?"

"Yes! I flew on your plane with Bob Hope, a few years ago. To Cleveland, wasn't it? For a charity golf tournament."

As we reminisced, that voice inside me whispered, "Tell him about the cookbook!"

We kept talking about this and that. Again the voice urged, "Tell him about the cookbook!" So I did. I told him about Brennan's diabetes and the cookbook, and how I had everything ready, but hadn't been able to find anyone to underwrite the project.

Ben said, "How much to you need?"

As nonchalantly as I could, I said, "About $40,000."

"I'll give you ten. Come on. Let's go out to the lobby. I've got some friends here tonight and this is Texas."

I left Houston with $17,500 to underwrite the project. A door had opened. Within four weeks, we had $42,500 pledged to pay for printing *The Days of Our Lives Celebrity Cookbook*, Volume I.

After ten months of trying to find sponsors, the money started flowing just after "Expect a Miracle" showed up in my dressing room. I tried to think of a rational explanation for the juxtaposition of that card and seeing Ben Rogers. Someone must have placed it there, yet they couldn't have known I'd see Ben the next day and that he'd be so generous. And what about that voice in my head telling me what to say? Those questions were the beginning of a life-changing inner journey, but that's another story for another book.

The Days of Our Lives Celebrity Cookbook was a big success. We sold out the first printing of 50,000 copies. Each copy was given as a gift in exchange for a minimum $10 donation to JDRF. We had an amazing amount of support: free advertising in *Good Housekeeping*, *Bon Appetit*, *Architectural Digest*, and *Newsweek*. We kept our expenses low: volunteers collected the mail, filled the orders. We printed another 50,000 copies of

Volume I and began work on Volume II. It was published in 1983 and sold another 50,000 copies.

I got another idea. I hadn't recorded an album in several years, so I decided to form a record company and produce an album as another fundraiser for JDRF. Another friend from Texas stepped forward to help, talking an acquaintance into underwriting the project titled "A Shot in the Dark." (The title song didn't have anything to do with insulin injections or the fact that trying to be a one-person record company was a bit risky, it was just a song I liked. It wasn't until I saw those words on the album cover that I recognized the pun.)

Between 1981 and 1985, the two cookbooks and the album raised close to one million dollars for diabetes research. It was an extraordinary time for all of us with the Los Angeles Chapter of JDRF. Those projects initiated my involvement in the world of diabetes research and care.

Tattered and stained, the "Expect a Miracle" card spent almost a year in the bottom of my travel bag before I noticed it. By then, I understood why I shouldn't throw it away. I framed it many years ago and it still graces my office wall. It reminds me of how benevolent life can be. I now know it's okay to expect a miracle, even in the face of seemingly insurmountable odds.

All the strategies of caring for diabetes involve keeping the blood sugar levels at normal as much as possible . . .

chapter two

a short course on diabetes

Diabetes is a complex metabolic disease. The two most common forms of diabetes are Type 1 and Type 2. There is also a new type of diabetes identified as Type 1.5, plus gestational diabetes that can occur during pregnancy.

No matter what type of diabetes a person has, the result is the same: too much sugar in the blood. The pancreas, a vital organ in your body, contains beta cells that produce insulin. Insulin is like a key that unlocks the door to each cell so that it can be nourished. Insulin also aids fat storage, as well as the manufacture of protein in the muscles.

When we eat food, it's digested and broken down into glucose, a simple form of sugar that then enters the bloodstream. Normally, the pancreas responds to an increase in blood glucose by releasing insulin. If there isn't enough insulin present, the glucose can't enter the cells. As excess glucose builds up in the blood, the kidneys try to excrete it in the urine. Sugar takes a lot of water with it when it leaves the body. That's why my son was so thirsty, drinking so much water, and was wetting the bed.

✦ ✦ ✦

type 1

Type 1 affects about ten percent of all cases of diabetes. It is most commonly diagnosed before age thirty and is also known as "juvenile diabetes." (Not "junior" diabetes, as I have heard people say.) With Type 1, the body no longer produces sufficient insulin because it has destroyed its own insulin-producing beta cells in the pancreas. The body mistakenly targets the beta cells for destruction and then the immune system attacks them as if they were foreign invaders. Researchers have discovered that this happens due to a combination of genetic factors combined with immune system malfunction triggered by viral infection. Environmental factors and stress are also suspected as triggering mechanisms. Once this destruction occurs, the missing insulin needs to be replaced by injection.

This describes what happened to Brennan. He was born with a genetic predisposition to develop Type 1. Six weeks before diagnosis, he had chicken pox. It's most likely that his body had been slowly attacking his beta cells for months or even years, and the chicken pox virus prompted a final assault which destroyed enough remaining beta cells to produce diabetes—higher than normal levels of glucose in the blood. At that point he needed injected insulin to stay healthy. Because insulin is a hormone, it cannot be taken orally, because stomach enzymes break it down.

type 2

Type 2 is known as non-insulin dependent or "maturity-onset" diabetes. It occurs most often in adults, but also occurs in overweight children. It's the most common form of diabetes, affecting 90% of all cases. In Type 2, the pancreas may be producing insulin, but either it's not enough to meet the body's needs or the body has become insulin resistant, no longer capable of using its insulin efficiently. Because of obesity, Type 2 has reached epidemic proportions in the United States and is on the rise.

Type 2 can usually be controlled through diet, exercise and oral medications, but can also require insulin injections. Oral medications taken for Type 2 are not a form of insulin. These are drugs that help the body use the insulin it already has or encourage it to produce more. Sometimes the oral drugs aren't enough. Forty percent of those with Type 2 eventually require insulin.

We don't know the exact cause of Type 2 diabetes. Many factors contribute to its occurrence. A person's risk increases significantly if she is obese, has a family history of diabetes, had diabetes during pregnancy, and is African American, Hispanic American, or Native American. Diabetes can also be caused by pancreatic and hormonal disorders, cystic fibrosis, Down's syndrome, congenital rubella syndrome, and in people undergoing drug therapy in which steroids such as Prednisone are used.

gestational diabetes

A woman can develop what is called "gestational" diabetes during the course of pregnancy. Some pregnant women have trouble metabolizing sugar. It's very important to properly manage gestational diabetes and keep the blood sugar levels normal to avoid complications for the mother and baby. That's why a pregnant woman under adequate prenatal care will have her urine checked for sugar at each doctor visit.

If a woman continues to have elevated blood sugars after pregnancy, the diagnosis is then Type 1 or Type 2 diabetes, or glucose intolerance. Even when the blood sugar returns to normal after pregnancy, there is an increased risk for Type 2 diabetes.

impaired glucose tolerance

With this problem, the body's response to sugar in the blood is impaired, but it hasn't yet become diabetes. This condition can be diagnosed using a glucose tolerance test. Although they don't usually present the classic diabetes symptoms, people who have it have the same problems with blood sugar levels as those with Type 2. People with IGT are twenty times more likely to develop diabetes. The U.S. Department of Health and Human services estimates that 40% of all U.S. adults between the ages of 40-74 years old are pre-diabetic, but very few know it. Half of the people who have IGT will eventually develop diabetes.

It's possible to prevent Type 2 diabetes in people who have IGT. In recent years, scientific studies have been performed all over the world to determine if increased physical activity or eating more carefully could indeed reduce the risk of developing diabetes. The results are encouraging. Recent studies conducted in Finland found that people with IGT who began a program of moderate exercise, healthier eating, and modest weight loss (just seven percent of their total body weight) reduced their risk of developing diabetes by fifty-eight percent.

type 1.5

There used to be only Type 1, Type 2, and gestational diabetes to talk about, but now there's a new kid in town: Type 1.5 diabetes. It's not well known in popular medical literature and it surprises physicians and patients alike when it happens. It shows up after age twenty-five and starts out acting like Type 2 diabetes.

For people with Type 1.5, their blood sugar levels may appear to be under control, but in a few months or years blood glucose levels increase and ketones appear in the urine. (Ketones are a by-product of the body burning fat for fuel.) The patient becomes dehydrated and begins losing weight. At this point oral medications are no longer sufficient and injected insulin is needed.

The difficulty in diagnosing it is that it can occur in slender individuals who exercise regularly and eat healthy foods. Dr. Tim's clinic has a sixty-year-old woman who recently developed Type 1.5. Some specialists call Type 1.5 "latent autoimmune diabetes of adulthood" or LADA.

diabesity

Until recently, Type 2 was most often diagnosed in people over thirty-five who had strong hereditary factors for the disease. If a person of average weight for their body type gets Type 2, it's hereditary factors that are at work. Some people with hereditary factors can avoid Type 2 by staying slim and exercising. Some cannot.

Yet even if there is no diabetes in the family, Type 2 looms as an ever-present possibility for people who are significantly overweight. Medical research has proven that there is a direct relationship between the severe overweight condition of many of our country's citizens and the 33 percent increase in diabetes in America in the last decade. Noted researcher and clinician Dr. Cal Ezrin has been working in the diabetes field for over fifty years and notes, "Most of the increase in diabetes is correlated with the increased prevalence of obesity. One of the most alarming things is seeing Type 2 diabetes among children as young as ten."

I remember when Type 2 diabetes in children was unknown. Doctors acknowledge that some children may develop it through genetic inheritance, but inheritance alone does not account for the epidemic we're seeing. Recent studies testify to the relationship of obesity and Type 2 in children. The faculty at Arkansas Children's Hospital studied medical diagnoses from 1988 to 1995 and found that 96 percent of the children with Type 2 diabetes were overweight. Another study at a Cincinnati children's hospital found that 92 percent of Type 2 adolescents were overweight.

Dr. Ezrin feels the word "diabesity" accurately describes the relationship between obesity and diabetes. He notes that he was not the first one to use this term. He told me, "Years ago, Professor of Medicine Ethan Sims at the University of Vermont wrote about it because he recognized the association between the disease and obesity."

busy fat

We think of fat as a passive thing. When I imagine lard or blubber, I see it just hanging around, perhaps jiggling a bit. Yet underneath that quiet Clark Kent exterior, it's a busy place. Fat is a chemical factory.

Dr. Ezrin explains: "If you gain fifteen or twenty pounds, for whatever reason, that fat generates an insulin antagonist. Researchers don't agree on what exactly it is, but it is a chemical that acts as a hormone and causes your cells to resist insulin."

Theoretically, the more fat there is, the greater the insulin resistance. The body tries to overcome the insulin resistance by producing more insulin. When an overweight person needs more insulin than she or he can produce, diabetes develops. Its symptoms include excessive thirst, excessive urination, unexplained weight loss, fatigue, blurred vision, sores and cuts that do not heal, and numbness or tingling in feet or hands. Or, strangely enough, there may not be any symptoms.

It's possible to reverse the symptoms of diabetes through loss of excess weight and lifestyle changes. A group of Australian Aborigines had "come to town" from the Outback, adopted the city lifestyle and food choices, and then developed Type 2 diabetes. When they returned home to their nomadic ways, eating less and walking every day, blood sugar levels improved and, in some cases, they no longer qualified as having diabetes. They basically "cured" themselves of diabetes. I'm not suggesting that you move to the Aussie bush land, but exercise and healthy food choices are essential factors in reversing diabetes. Conversely, many people with Type 2 who don't address needed lifestyle changes eventually require insulin injections.

No matter what type of diabetes or pre-diabetes condition you have, your cells are not getting as much glucose (sugar) as they need because you don't have enough insulin to support your metabolism. Insulin is the key that unlocks the doors of the cells to let energy-giving glucose in. If there isn't enough insulin, glucose can't enter the cells and builds up in the blood, causing high blood sugar. High blood sugar damages your body, slowly and certainly. All the strategies of caring for diabetes involve keeping the blood sugar levels at normal levels as much as possible through the strategies of proper nutrition, exercise, and appropriate medication.

*Diabetes demands
attention. It requires
more than most other
diseases, a high level
of self-care.*

chapter three

yeah, team!

I have two concerts next week, so I know I must spend some time preparing for those performances. I take time to exercise my voice each day so it will be ready for the demands of a two-hour rehearsal and a two-hour show. I sing through the songs so that the lyrics will flow easily when the moment comes. I do this because I know that my happiest moments are when I sing freely, the voice open and relaxed, the song's meaning and feeling coming straight from my heart. I don't want any obstacles to get in the way of giving my best. By trial and error, I have learned one certainty: there is no freedom without discipline.

The quality of my performance will also be the result of a team effort. My singing teacher has taught me good vocal habits and knowledgeable use of my voice. My musical director and musicians support me with feeling and expertise. A designer with an eye for how I look best created my gown.

So it is with diabetes: your being free to live your life without obstacles (complications) will be the result of discipline—daily attention to your body's needs—and the knowledgeable support of a good team.

Dr. Ken Quickel calls diabetes "a team sport." Ken is the former CEO of the Joslin Diabetes Center in Boston and spent most of his professional life in the diabetes arena. A few years ago, he was diagnosed with Type 2, so he knows diabetes from both sides of the desk.

Dr. Quickel says, "Diabetes requires the knowledge of many different people to get the best control of it within each individual's lifestyle. The captain of the team is the patient and she's got to become the best player on the team. She has to know everything there is to know about her own diabetes, be a student of the disease. It's the moment-to-moment care of diabetes that makes the difference. It's what happens on Saturday afternoon after a two-mile walk in the park and you're having an insulin reaction or what you do when you're out to dinner and the *crème brulée* shows up. Those are decisions you make on your own."

I agree, and to help the captain make good choices, the captain needs a playbook from an expert coach and staff. So, who should be on your diabetes team?

Ideally, your team would include:

+ Your primary care physician who practices general medicine, treating a wide range of medical problems. If this doctor will be caring for your diabetes, he should have significant experience and interest in treating diabetes, and should not be hesitant to refer you to diabetes specialist. Preferably, he should have a diabetes educator on staff.

+ An endocrinologist or diabetologist with a significant Type 2 practice that has specialized training and experience in diabetes.

+ A certified diabetes educator (C.D.E.) or diabetes nurse educator (D.N.E.) who trains you in daily diabetes management, answers your questions, helps with problems, and supports and guides required lifestyle changes.

+ A registered dietitian (R.D.) who assesses your nutritional needs and tailors a meal plan that accounts for your budget, preferences, and lifestyle.

+ An exercise physiologist who assesses your body's exercise needs and designs a program that helps control your blood sugar levels.

✦ An ophthalmologist who will monitor your eyes to detect and treat problems early so you can avoid diabetic eye damage.

✦ A podiatrist who will help you take great care of your feet and avoid complications.

your diabetes doctor

As Dr. Tim noted in his personal story, diabetes is a very complicated disease and requires expertise and commitment of time. You'll receive the most knowledgeable care from either a primary care physician or an endocrinologist who is an expert in diabetes and treats many Type 2 patients. The problem is that some insurance plans limit access to specialists and diabetes education programs. If that's the case, your primary care physician, working in concert with a certified diabetes educator, can provide good overall direction and a personally tailored plan.

Even though you may do well under this arrangement, it's advisable to see a diabetes specialist for a yearly check-up to be certain nothing is missed. If there isn't a diabetes specialist in your community, your doctor and diabetes educator can help you locate one in a neighboring city. Establishing a relationship with the specialist who will be familiar with your needs can be especially helpful in the case of an illness or emergency. You can then call that doctor for a phone consultation and know you're getting additional expert advice.

At the same time, don't overlook the importance of your primary care doctor. One of the problems of receiving specialty care is that people forget to do some of the things that primary care doctors do. When female patients only see specialists, they tend to get fewer Pap smears or tend to have their mammograms further apart, because the focus is on one disease and one course of treatment. For recommendations of good diabetes specialists, you can call your local American Diabetes Association (ADA) chapter or talk with your educator and those who have diabetes. You can call your county Medical Society or go to your public library and check the *Directory of Medical Specialists*.

In the early days of your diagnosis, don't be shy about calling your health care professional when you have questions. Diabetes is new to you and you deserve help and support. Another strategy is to partner with a diabetes mentor, someone who's had diabetes for several years and can provide insight based on personal experience. Your mentor may offer good ideas you can talk over with your doctor or educator.

your diabetes educator and dietitian

Your diabetes educator is an essential member of your team. Few doctors can devote the time it takes to empower you to care for your diabetes. A Certified Diabetes Educator (C.D.E.) specializes in diabetes management and can spend the hours it will take to turn you into an expert.

Usually, a doctor specializing in diabetes has a team that includes a diabetes educator and dietitian. Sometimes the diabetes educator is also a R.D., Registered Dietitian and has passed a national credentialing exam. Your educator may also have earned a Master of Science degree (M.S.) or Master of Arts degree (M.A.) and in some states, might also be licensed as an L.D., a Licensed Dietitian. So you might find an educator and dietitian who is identified as Susan Smith, M.S., R.D., L.D., C.D.E.

Your diabetes educator (and dietitian, if you have a separate person as that) will spend time helping you understand the aspects of your care regimen: your food plan to help stabilize your blood sugar, a weight loss program, if you need one, and an exercise regimen, if you aren't working with an exercise physiologist. All of these strategies are designed to bring your blood sugar into the normal range, so that you can avoid the complications of diabetes. If your doctor doesn't have a diabetes educator in his office, contact your local American Diabetes Association or the American Association of Diabetes Educators. (Addresses and phone numbers are listed in the Resources Section.) Your diabetes educator is an essential member of your diabetes team. Don't have diabetes without one!

✦ ✦ ✦

your eye specialist

You will need a yearly examination by an ophthalmologist trained in diabetes care. If you don't have an ophthalmologist in your community, you may be able to find an optometrist, identified by O.D. after his name, who is familiar with diabetes. Your exam should include a dilated eye exam so that the doctor can look at the back of the eye for any changes in the retina. With Type 1 diabetes, the first exam is usually scheduled five years after diagnosis. Yet because Type 2 diabetes often goes undetected for several years, it's advisable to have a dilated eye exam soon after your initial diagnosis.

In recent years, new equipment has improved the gathering of information about the health of the eyes. One of these technological advances is a fundus camera. It takes a picture of the retina. These pictures, along with a letter detailing the results of your eye exam, can be sent to your physician.

Dr. Lloyd Aiello of Joslin Diabetes Center had a hand in developing laser surgery for diabetic eye disease. Dr. Aiello has devised a new diagnostic tool: digital imaging techniques. It's not yet widely available, but Dr. Aiello hopes it will be soon. These techniques produce a three dimensional picture of the inside of the eye. They're fast, easy, and don't require the eye to be dilated. The images provide detailed information about subtle changes in the eye. The sooner these changes are found, the more likely they can be effectively treated. Dr. Aiello states it is possible to save 98 percent of severe vision loss that occurs in people with diabetes. Yet diabetes is still the leading cause of new blindness in this country. Why? Because too many people with diabetes don't go for a yearly eye exam with an ophthalmologist trained to see the early warning signs. Please don't put off having your eyes checked.

your podiatrist

A podiatrist is a foot and ankle surgeon who has special knowledge about diabetes and its effects on circulation to your extremities. If you have problems with your feet and legs, your doctor may have you consult a podiatrist to get expert advice.

a mentor

Once you have your health care professional team assembled, you may want to add one more member: a mentor who is taking good care of his or her diabetes. No one understands diabetes better than someone who is also living with it. Let your diabetes educator or doctor know you're interested in connecting with a mentor. You might also join the local diabetes support group or American Diabetes Association chapter and connect with someone there. It's essential that you understand what diabetes is and how it works in your body. You could buy a really good book about diabetes and read it. (Oh yes, you're already doing that.) Once you think you've ready, talk with your educator or diabetes mentor and explain diabetes to them. Then ask if you got it right.

Keep in touch with the latest developments in diabetes care and research through magazines and newsletters. When you begin to feel confident in your understanding and caring for your diabetes, you might offer to become a mentor to someone who has recently been diagnosed.

your exam should include:

✦ Weight
✦ Blood pressure
✦ Urine analysis
✦ Blood glucose *(taken at the office)*
✦ Comparison of your blood testing monitor *with lab results for meter accuracy*
✦ Foot examination—*Your doctor should look at your feet every time you have a checkup. Take your shoes off and ask the doctor to check them if he doesn't offer.*
✦ Hemoglobin A1c *(glycosylated hemoglobin or fructosamine)*
✦ A discussion of your blood test diary and noted trends

your exam

Ideally, you should have an examination every three to four months. Remind your doctor at the time of your exam about important aspects of your care. It's a good idea to create a calendar for your doctor's appointments and book them well in advance, every three months, plus your yearly eye and dental exams. Write down questions as they arise and take that list with you to your appointments. And ask them! Write down the answers. Your doctor will be pleased that you care about how well you're doing.

If you need your doctor's referral for an eye exam, tell him, "I haven't had my eyes checked for ten months. It's time for me to see an ophthalmologist in the next two months."

The Joslin Diabetes Center recommends that your yearly exam with your diabetes doctor include all of the above, plus the following:

✦ A complete physical examination, including assessment of your blood pressure, total cholesterol level, plus LDL and HDL levels and triglycerides.
✦ Urine test for protein (microalbumin) to monitor your kidneys
✦ C-reactive protein test (CRP) for arterial inflammation
✦ Thyroid function test (TSH)
✦ Testing for blood chemistries and blood counts, including electrolytes, blood urea nitrogen (BUN), and creatinine

What are your exam goals?

✦ Blood pressure—below 130/80 mg/dl
✦ Total cholesterol—below 200
✦ LDL cholesterol—below 100 mg/dl
✦ HDL cholesterol—above 40 mg/dl men; above 50 mg/dl in women
✦ Triglycerides—below 150 mg/dl
✦ Microalbumin test—no protein in the urine
✦ C-reactive protein (CRP)—below 3.0

Add to the above the need for a yearly eye exam and dental exam. Seems like a lot, doesn't it? Yet your life and health are worth all that TLC. In some cases, you may not get all this care unless you ask for it. It's important that you're a well-informed patient who knows what ought to be done and when. One expert told me, "If everyone with diabetes were well trained to be an expert, we could cut the complication rate in half."

In the Resources for Readers section, we've provided a chart for you to take to the doctor's office to keep track of all these tests and numbers.

blood pressure

So, what are these tests and what do they mean? Let's start with blood pressure. Monitoring blood pressure levels is very important to a person with diabetes. Your objective is to keep your blood pressure in the "normal range." By the way, there's a new "normal."

Until recently, normal blood pressure was defined as less than 140 systolic and less than 90 diastolic (140/90). New guidelines issued in 2003 by the National Heart, Lung, and Blood Institute have lowered the bar. Normal is now defined as less than 120/80. Because damage to arteries begins at fairly low blood pressure levels, a new "pre-hypertension" level was added, from 120–139 over 80–89 (120/80 to 139/89). Studies have shown that the risk of death from heart disease and stroke begins to rise at blood pressure levels as low as 115/75.

For someone on a blood pressure treatment plan, it is recommended that levels be less than 140/90. For those with diabetes and kidney disease, the recommendation is lower than 130/80. There are good reasons for this. High blood pressure, diabetes, and kidney disease work together to make each even more dangerous.

If your blood pressure is above these guidelines, pay attention to the warning your body is giving you. There is much you can do to change the situation. In a report by the Joint National Committee on *Prevention, Detection, Evaluation, and Treatment of High Blood Pressure*, lifestyle changes were very effective in decreasing blood pressure. They reported that weight loss could lower systolic pressure by 5 to 20 points per 22 pounds lost. Eating a diet high in fruits and vegetables and low in fat can reduce blood pressure by 8 to 14 points. Limiting salt to 2400mg per day caused a 2 to 8 point reduction and limiting alcohol to no more than two drinks per day caused a reduction of 2 to 4 points. Thirty minutes of daily exercise reduced blood pressure by 4 to 9 points.

My friend Hilda recently went on a ten-day health retreat. When she left for the retreat, she had high blood pressure and was twenty pounds overweight. While she was there, she exercised each day, ate mostly fruits, whole grains, and vegetables, drank no alcohol, and took yoga and meditation classes. In ten days her blood pressure dropped 25 points. Both Hilda and her doctor were amazed. Lifestyle changes can indeed improve your blood pressure as much as medication.

cholesterol

You want your total cholesterol to be below 200, but don't be satisfied with only knowing that number. There are two types of cholesterol: LDL and HDL. LDL, low-density lipoprotein, is considered "bad," because it's deposited in the arteries. HDL, high-density lipoprotein, is considered "good" because it sweeps excess cholesterol from the arteries and carries it back to the liver. So you want to have low numbers for the LDL (think *less desirable*) and higher numbers for HDL (think *highly desirable!*). Your goal is to keep "good" HDL cholesterol above 40mg/dl for men and 50mg/dl for women; and keep your "bad" LDL cholesterol below 100mg/dl. Ideal LDL cholesterol is below 80.

Saturated fats (animal fats and hydrogenated oils) raise the level of LDL and make you more susceptible to clogged arteries. Unsaturated fat is thought to help prevent heart and blood vessel disease by lowering LDL cholesterol and raising the level of HDL cholesterol.

triglycerides

Because triglyceride levels above 200 mg/dl are associated with increased risk of heart attack and stroke, you want to know your level. Triglycerides are a type of fat storage system, and higher than normal blood sugar will increase your triglyceride levels. Since diabetes already increases your risk of heart attack, work closely with your doctor to use exercise, healthy eating, and medication, if necessary, to keep your level of triglycerides below 100mg/dl.

microalbumin test

This test detects protein, also known as albumin, in the urine and is an important indicator of how your kidneys are handling diabetes. When a person is first diagnosed, it's a good idea to have this test done, either with a spot sample of urine (the easy way) or with a twenty-four-hour urine test. The kidneys do not normally lose any protein. If they do, it's a sign of kidney damage. The sooner it is discovered, the better. New drugs known as ACE Inhibitors or ARB (angiotensin receptor blockers) can help lower blood pressure in the kidneys and limit further kidney damage.

c-reactive protein (crp)

CRP is a relatively new blood test that measures inflammation in your heart and brain arteries. Studies have shown that half the people with heart attacks or strokes have normal cholesterol, but high C-reactive protein. One Harvard University study of 28,000 women showed that a high CRP is more predictive of a heart attack than LDL cholesterol.

The liver produces C-reactive protein in response to inflammation and poor lifestyle. It causes monocytes, white blood cells, to burrow into the artery walls and cause plaque buildup. One doctor calls CRP "the truth serum for your lifestyle."

Your CRP should be below 3.0 and 1.0 is ideal. If your CRP is high, stop smoking (if you do), start exercising, and eat a really healthy diet with fresh fruits and vegetables and healthy fats. Add a tablespoon or two of freshly ground flaxseed to each meal. These lifestyle changes are proven methods of decreasing CRP levels. Statin and TZD medications may decrease your arterial inflammation, but may not lower your CRP level. It takes about six months for lifestyle changes to change your CRP, so ask your doctor to schedule a CRP blood test twice a year.

✦ ✦ ✦

hemoglobin a1c

A lot of money has been spent on diabetes research in the past few decades. We no longer have to let diabetes do the unchecked damage it's done in the past. You have a really good chance of living a healthy, unobstructed life with diabetes, if you become a warrior. A warrior learns all she can about her foe's ways and then chooses her weapon carefully.

Your primary weapon in challenging diabetes is the Hemoglobin A1c, also known as the HbA1c. Dr. Tim thinks it's so important that his license plate reads: "HBA1C." This test measures the amount of excess glucose that clings to the red blood cells from the previous ninety days. That's why you should get an HbA1c every three or four months. I've spoken with too many people who either don't know if their doctor does an HbA1c or aren't sure what the reading is.

Health professionals once believed that keeping your blood sugar levels tightly controlled and close to normal didn't really make a difference. They thought that diabetes itself damaged the body, not the higher-than-normal blood sugar levels. A ten-year national study called The Diabetes Control and Complications Trial (DCCT) proved they were wrong. The DCCT clearly demonstrated that carefully controlled blood sugar could reduce eye, kidney, and nerve damage up to 76 percent, 39 percent, and 60, percent respectively. At the time the trial was completed, the desired HbA1c level for adults was said to be 7.1 or below. Now, 6.5 or below is considered the ideal level.

To understand what the HbA1c means in terms of your blood sugar levels, take the number of your HbA1c and subtract 2. If your result is 6.5, subtract 2 and you get 4.5. Then multiply that number by 30 and you get your average blood sugar for the last ninety days. So 4.5 x 30 = 135. Even though that's above the normal range of 80 to 120, an HbA1c of 6.5 diminishes your risk of complications. When you lower your HbA1c, you decrease your chances of damage from diabetes.

A patient of Dr. Tim's, John, has recently begun to understand how important a predictor of complications the HbA1c can be. He never believed he had to make lifestyle changes to take care of his diabetes. His HbA1c was 12.2. Putting that into our formula: 12.2—2 = 10.2 x 30 = 306 average blood sugar. His HbA1c was telling him a story he refused to hear.

Then John started having small strokes. Diabetes finally got John's attention. John's son, Willie, moved in with his parents and took charge of the shopping and cooking. Willie, known in the family as "Whole Wheat Willie," is a health food enthusiast who now has his parents on a walking program. He accompanies his dad to doctors appointments and takes notes. He has also attended diabetes education classes to learn how to prevent further problems. John is now on track for good control of his diabetes. He's lucky to have a son like Willie.

Please get an HbA1c done every three to four months. Your doctor may not tell you the result. ASK. Don't let the doctor tell you, "Oh, it's fine" You decide if it's fine. If your doctor accepts too high a reading, he will not suffer the complications. If your HbA1c is 6.5 or lower, you're doing well. If it's higher, ask your doctor or diabetes educator for a blood sugar control tune up.

smoking

There is one more important task for you and your doctor to achieve. If you smoke, do everything you can to stop. Get your doctor to prescribe the latest stop-smoking aids. Go to a support group. Form a "Circle of Friends" (a national campaign) to encourage you. Chew gum, eat carrots, take up meditation, practice yoga, run a marathon. Whatever it takes, listen to Nike: "Just do it."

Why should you stop smoking? For a person with diabetes, carbon monoxide from inhaled smoke sticks to red blood cells. It prevents them from carrying oxygen, and:

✦   One cigarette per day constricts the blood vessels for up to twenty-four hours so they can't get as much blood to eyes, skin, etc. The same thing happens if you breathe in second-hand smoke.
✦   You need more insulin if you smoke.
✦   Smoking seriously increases your danger of leg/foot ulcers or infections, which may lead to the loss of a foot or leg. Smoking increases your risk of blindness, impotence, kidney failure, heart disease, and stroke.

Diabetes is very hard on the systems of your body. A recent study revealed that 22 percent of Americans with diabetes smoke. Diabetes causes problems with blood vessels, from the smallest to the largest, and smoking enhances the danger of complications. Smoking provokes constriction of the arteries similar to plunging your hand into a bucket of ice water.

If you're ready to quit smoking, enlist the help of your health care provider. Consider using several strategies at once. The combination of counseling and the use of trans-dermal nicotine patches has been shown to be much more effective than trying to quit on your own.

perspective: being (a) patient

I looked up the word "patient" in my old friend *Webster's* and was treated to these definitions: "The will or ability to wait and endure without complaint; steadiness, endurance, or perseverance in performing a task," and "A person receiving care or treatment." Sounds like diabetes to me. (Although some of us wouldn't qualify for the "without complaint" aspect of that definition.)

Perhaps you've heard the prayer, "Lord, give me patience . . . and give it to me now." Heaven knows, having diabetes requires patience. The practice of patience begins when you are first diagnosed and you are led through the details of what diabetes is and what you will now have to do to take care of your body. It can feel overwhelming.

Diabetes slows down your life. That's not necessarily a bad thing, but it may require shifting gears from your previous pace. There's more to do and more to think about. You don't just jump out of bed and start your day. You stop and test your blood sugar—check in with your body to see how it's doing. You don't just eat whenever you like. You pay more attention to when you eat and what you eat. You test your blood sugar when needed, and take your medication or injections. (There's the "steadiness" part.)

You do learn patience, especially with your inability to get your body to always respond the way you'd like. Sometimes your blood sugars are in the desired range. Sometimes they're not. Since you're in this for the long haul, you know that one undesirable blood sugar does not mean too much.

So you practice patience and work toward the next time. (That's the "perseverance" and "endurance" part).

Which brings us to the second part of the definition, the part about being a patient. I sometimes wonder if this aspect of "patient" comes from the long waits we often endure in the doctor's office. Yet there's more to being a patient than being patient. What kind of a patient are you? Are you a passive one, enduring and persevering? Do you only pay close attention to your diabetes the week before your doctor visit?

Or are you the team leader, working with your diabetes professionals? Diabetes requires, more than most other diseases, a high level of self-care. Your commitment to your own health and your understanding of the way diabetes affects your body determines the quality of your care and will impact the quality of your life.

Not long ago, there was a celebration at the Joslin Clinic in Syracuse, New York. The Cleveland brothers, Robert and Gerald, were honored at a presentation attended by doctors from Joslin Clinic in Boston and one hundred friends and family members. Their former doctor, the father of their current doctor, flew in from North Carolina to attend. Robert was recognized as the only person living with diabetes for seventy-nine years. Gerald is close behind that record at seventy-two years.

Take a moment: Can you imagine yourself twenty, thirty, forty years from now? What does that look like? Imagine being at a celebration of your many years of living with diabetes, surrounded by your family and friends, along with your diabetes care team members. Imagine them all feeling pride and respect for the example you've set, for how diligently you worked to come to that day. See yourself with your body and all its attendants—eyes, limbs, inner organs—healthy and vital. Is there a pencil or pen close by right now? Use it to finish this sentence:

Years from now, I see myself healthy and feeling _____

_____

_____

_____

The realization of that day begins now. To achieve that goal, I am willing to:

❒ Learn what diabetes is and how it affects my body.

❒ Learn why I perform each aspect of my care regimen.

❒ Learn what a glycosylated hemoglobin (HbA1c) test is and have one done every three months.

❒ Work with my team to keep my HbA1c at or below 6.5.

❒ Get my eyes examined every year by an ophthalmologist or qualified optometrist.

❒ Have yearly screenings for signs of complications.

❒ Connect with others who have diabetes, either by seeking or giving support.

❒ Be a role model for others by taking excellent care of myself.

❒ Keep up with the latest diabetes research and product developments.

. . . laughter can increase your tolerance to pain, lower your risk of heart attack, reduce your levels of stress hormones, and boost your immune system.

chapter four

what a difference a day makes

Deborah was diagnosed with diabetes on her ninth birthday. She's lived with insulin injections and blood testing for more than forty years. After all this time, she is free from diabetes complications and determined to stay that way. I think the secret to her success has been her perspective. From the day she was diagnosed, her family's mission was to learn everything they could about diabetes and share their knowledge with others. Because of their attitude, Deborah decided that if she had to have a disease, diabetes wasn't so bad.

Deborah tells the story: "I remember lying on the bed one morning. It was months after I'd been diagnosed, and Mother was going to give me the injection in my hip. I turned my head and asked her, 'When will my shots be over?'

"She hesitated. 'Well . . . when a cure is found.'

"I said, 'I really do believe they'll find a cure. Don't you?'

"She said, 'Yes, I do. Until then, Deborah, it's very important that you take good care of yourself.'"

Deborah's success is also attributable to Granny Whitaker's motto, "Every invitation is a command." Deborah has taken it to heart and doesn't want anything to ever prevent her from having an adventure. She says, "Long before my diabetes was diagnosed, there was a word I did not like. That word is NO. I will do everything and anything to avoid hearing that word. I think that's why I'm so disciplined. I never wanted to hear, 'You can't do that because you're a diabetic.' I've wanted to prove to people that I can do anything my heart desires."

Deborah calls her diabetes paraphernalia "my treasures." When she was a counselor at diabetes camp in the mid-1970s, there was a researcher at the camp who was really scaring the campers about the complications of diabetes. She didn't like calling diabetes supplies "life support," as the researcher had sternly described them. She wanted her campers to look at their supplies in a positive way, so she suggested that their supplies were special treasures and that if they kept them close and dear, the frightening complications the doctor warned about would never happen to them. She's called her diabetes supplies "treasures" ever since. This chapter is about the treasures that will help you live a long and healthy life . . . with diabetes.

your daily treasures

Some people take on the task of "daily treasures" eagerly. Dr. Tim's patient, Karen, discovered she had Type 2 diabetes when she went to the hospital for an angiogram. Before the procedure, they tested her blood glucose level: it was 300. Fortunately, Karen is obsessive-compulsive. She religiously checks her blood glucose and has made necessary lifestyle changes. Karen feels she has a good reason to take care of herself: a new granddaughter in the family. Karen wants to be around to enjoy her granddaughter for many years to come. For Karen, diabetes was a wake-up call. She says, "Now that I have diabetes, I give myself permission to take care of me. I take time to eat well and exercise, and to perform blood tests every day."

When you've been diagnosed with diabetes, your doctor or educator will instruct you to check your blood sugar. *Reality alert*: If your doctor tells you that he'll test you in the office so you don't have to do it at home, don't accept that as good enough care. I've met people with Type 2 who don't test themselves every day. They say they have "borderline" diabetes. That's like being a little bit pregnant. Don't buy it. You either have higher than normal blood sugar or you don't. Just as with blood pressure, any reading over the high end of normal (120mg/dl) carries potential for damage. Knowing how your blood sugar is reacting to food and activity each day is essential. Just because you don't know about your reading doesn't mean it won't affect you. Your doctor will not suffer the complications if your care is inadequate. You will.

Considering diabetes is more than two-thousand years old, home blood sugar monitoring is a fairly recent development. It's quite an improvement over the testing we used to do when Brennan was first diagnosed—urine testing. It measured how much excess sugar was spilling into the urine over a period of hours and was only an approximation of the actual blood sugar level.

I recall a story I heard from a parent about her son's first time at diabetes camp. A few of the kids were feeling frisky one morning and told their counselor that instead of doing individual urine tests, they would all pee in the barrel and she could average it out. That's a pretty good analogy for a urine test.

My son's doctor told me of adolescent patients who would dilute their urine with tap water to ensure negative results at the doctor's office. A fresh urine sample is quite warm, as it has just left the body. The doctor would stick his finger into the diluted sample and remark, "Either this is a mistake or you died a week ago."

Although testing your blood sugar several times a day may not be your idea of a trip to Disneyland, it's essential for your health and quality of life. My dentist says, "Only brush and floss the teeth you want to keep." So it is with diabetes: Only test and control your blood sugar levels if you want to keep your eyes and kidneys and feet and legs and heart and sexual function. Otherwise, don't pay any attention to this chapter.

becoming a chemist

When Brennan was diagnosed in 1979, I felt I was being asked to become a chemist. I had to know exactly how many units of insulin to load into a syringe. We were instructed to keep Brennan's blood sugar in the normal range as much as possible—between 80 and 120 mg/dl. There were different insulins: beef and pork, Regular and NPH, Lente and UltraLente. At first we did urine tests; then there was home blood glucose monitoring. We kept a diary of the results. We learned to test for ketones. We were taught how to use the "Exchange Diet": half a cup of this fruit is equal to 1/3 cup of that fruit. My brain was overloaded with details. I called the doctor and diabetes educator two or three times a day for weeks.

With Type 2 diabetes, there's still a lot to learn, but that's why you have this book in your hands. You may not have to take insulin injections, but whether you have Type 1 or Type 2, the other aspects of controlling blood sugar levels are basically the same. In addition to taking medication prescribed by your doctor, your most important daily task is testing your blood sugar.

Why? Your body is no longer able to perform the routine task of checking and adjusting the amount of sugar in your blood. That job is now yours. (Ah, for the good old days when it was an automatic process.) Testing at varying times will help you keep track of how your medication is working and how your eating and exercise patterns are affecting your levels. Even though your before-breakfast numbers look good, your lunchtime or night-time blood sugar levels may not be in the target range.

What is the target range? Ideally, your blood sugar should be 80 to 120mg/dl first thing in the morning and before meals. (The term "mg/dl" is a standard of measurement that means milligram per deciliter.) Two hours after meals, it's best if it's in the 140 to 160mg/dl range. At bedtime, it should be about 140mg/dl. Those may seem like difficult goals to achieve, but higher than normal blood sugar levels cause complications. Avoiding long-term complications is worth whatever effort it takes.

There are also short-term rewards. By testing, you can see your blood sugar level at any given moment. If it's low, it can be treated with some sugar-containing food. It can be embarrassing and scary to have a low blood sugar reaction in front of co-workers or strangers. The symptoms can range from sweating and shaking to unfortunate behavior. June Biermann and Barbara Toohey tell a story in one of their esteemed diabetes books about a meeting at their publisher's office. In the midst of a serious discussion, June began to swear, using some rather surprising words. Barbara reached into her purse and handed June some candy. June ate it and a few minutes later everything was back to normal. After the meeting, one of the attendees asked June, "You reward her when she talks like that?"

when to test

When should you test? Blood sugar testing is usually done first thing in the morning, before meals, two hours after you began eating a meal, at bedtime, during the night, and any time you feel "different."

If you're on insulin, you should test at least four times a day, before each meal and at bedtime. You should also spot-check your blood sugar two hours after meals during the week (that's called a post-prandial blood sugar) and before an exercise session. It's recommended that you test before you drive your car, as it can help you avoid a very low blood sugar that could lead to loss of consciousness. For a long time, my friend Jerry (who is on injected insulin) refused to test himself consistently. One night he lost consciousness due to low blood sugar and nearly drove off the side of a mountain. Now he tests.

If you're on oral medication, Dr. Tim recommends that you test twice a day. If you test only once, it's difficult to maintain control of your blood sugar, since you don't get enough information to help you make the best decisions. By testing both before a meal and two hours after you begin eating, you can learn how much your blood sugar increases with various foods. For instance, you might discover that beef increases your blood sugar more than chicken or a banana more than an apple.

Here's a suggested daily testing schedule from Dr. Tim:

- ✦ The first day, test before breakfast and two hours after breakfast.
- ✦ The next day, test before lunch and two hours after lunch.
- ✦ The third day, you can test before supper or two hours after supper and bedtime.
- ✦ Always test before driving a car and before exercising.

As you follow this schedule for a few weeks, patterns will emerge that help you see how your medication and food choices are balancing and where you need to make adjustments. You may find there are obstacles to testing your blood sugar as often as recommended. If you have Type 2 diabetes and are not using insulin, your insurance may not pay for more than one test strip daily. If this occurs, please purchase extra strips to monitor your blood sugar. It may stretch your budget, but care of your diabetes is not the place to cut corners.

If you suffer from anxiety or fear of testing, or there are physical or mental limitations that prevent you from testing yourself, you can have a family member learn to perform your testing ritual. The same is true if you have severe vision problems and aren't able to test your blood dependably. BIG WARNING! Don't be afraid to ask for help.

A few years ago, I interviewed a man named Bill. No one had helped Bill understand the damage diabetes can do. As Bill told me, "The doctor told me I had Type 2 Diabetes and had to go on a special diet. I tried to follow the diet, but like most people with diabetes, I did not follow it because it was too hard."

He also didn't test his blood sugar. Before too long, he began to lose his vision. Even then, he didn't seem to understand it was essential that he set high standards for his own care. When I asked Bill how his diabetes care was going, he admitted, "I do not test my blood sugar everyday. My wife will test it for me when I ask her to, but I just don't ask her because she has so much on her right now . . . writing checks for the bills, opening the mail, etc. I feel she has more of a load on her since my vision has become impaired." Two years later I heard from Bill. In spite of laser surgery, he was legally blind.

your daily diary

Why is it necessary to keep a record of your test results? For one thing, it helps you watch for patterns that indicate the effectiveness of your medication. A written record gives you information you and your doctor can use to adjust your medication and your overall exercise and food plan. It also gives you quick visual feedback about the way your daily schedule of food, exercise, and stress are affecting your control.

Sometimes the picture isn't very encouraging. Don't be dismayed. You and your doctor are trying to replicate an amazingly complex and elegant system created by a master intelligence. Just like relationships, you're not going to get it exactly right every time. Why is your blood sugar sometimes above the target range? The usual suspects are too much food and not enough exercise. It could also be that you're not taking enough insulin or oral medication. It may be that your emotions are running high with anger or stress, or you're getting sick with a fever or a urinary tract infection.

When there's an out of control reading or pattern, look and listen to what your diary is telling you. Thai food for dinner and the next morning's blood sugar is over the moon? Oops, Thai food is often high in sugar. You didn't know that? Next time you will. If you can't figure out what caused high readings, call your diabetes educator to help you piece together a high blood sugar's originating cause. Your diabetes mentor is also very valuable in this area, because he or she has had lots of experience with the causes of high readings.

Whatever the reason for the high reading, please remember that blood sugar control is not a moral issue. Some of us put so much pressure on ourselves to be perfect. One or more high blood sugar readings don't mean you failed some existential test. What matters most is your overall consistency. Your HbA1c numbers will tell the truth of your efforts.

In my first meeting with Brennan's diabetes educator, I was advised that test results are not "bad" or "good." Following her lead, I announced test results as high, low, or in target range. I'm sure the "Oh, that's good," slipped out occasionally, but I made a concerted effort not to call high blood sugar "bad." I tried to paint a high reading as a puzzle, "Let's see if we can figure out what happened."

Your daily diary is your personal diabetes educator. As you fill in information about all the elements that may have affected your blood sugar, you will get to know how your individual system reacts to certain foods, different types of exercise and your medication. Dr. Tim says that if you only write down the number, you won't remember all the things that could have affected it. It's like when you're moving and while packing a box, you say to yourself, "Oh, I don't have to label it. I'll remember what's in it." Fat chance.

your meter

The technology that supports home blood glucose monitoring is wonderfully simple. You place a drop of your blood on a strip or contact point and an electrical charge stimulated by the sugar in the blood gives a precise reading of your blood's sugar content at that moment. Self-monitoring is quick, easy, and almost painless. All the meters are accurate to within 15 percent of a venous blood test (blood your doctor takes from a vein).

Your insurer may direct which of the monitors they will pay for or your educator can give you a recommendation. It's important that the meter fits the ability of the person operating it. No matter where you buy your meter, have a trained professional teach you how to use it. Don't buy a meter at the local pharmacy or by mail order and begin to use it without your educator or pharmacist giving you a thorough demonstration.

There are more than thirty different glucose-monitoring systems. Some meters use a non-wipe technology to decrease the amount of extra work you do for cleanup. For people with limited vision, there's the Accucheck Verbal Voicemate meter. It tells you what to do next if you can't see the meter screen clearly. If you need tight glucose control for hours at a time, there is the Glucowatch Biographer. You wear it on your wrist and it records blood glucose every few minutes. It can be set with alarms to warn you of low blood sugar or excessively high blood sugar.

There's no one meter that's right for everyone. Dr. Tim's favorite is the Accucheck Compact, his nurse prefers the Ascensia Elite, and his diabetes educator's favorite is the Accucheck Advantage. The Resources for Readers section at the back of this book lists almost all the meters and their advantages, and the companies that manufacture them. Talk with your educator about which meter is best for you.

Because the current sensor technology doesn't permit you to read a test strip visually, it's a good idea to have a second meter. If your battery runs down or your meter breaks, you have no way of knowing your blood sugar. Also, don't throw away an old meter. Medical companies frequently have trade-ins or rebates for used meters. The drug companies offer this because if you're using their meter, you're buying their test strips. Each machine has its own brand of strips and the companies make a lot more money on the strips than they do on the meters.

Another important warning: don't use someone else's meter. Blood carries the risk of infecting others with HIV or hepatitis. Infection is possible when you come in contact with another person's blood, or when he or she is exposed to yours. Also, never share or handle lancets owned by somebody else.

how to: blood tests

Let's go through the blood-testing ritual. It's going to sound like a lot of instructions at first, but in a short time you'll be able to perform the whole routine in a few minutes.

Begin by washing your hands. Gather your lancet, automatic lancet device, meter, and appropriate test strip. If you're opening a new vial of test strips, compare the code number on your meter to the code number on the vial of strips. If they don't match, follow the manufacturer's instructions to change the code number.

Next, turn the meter on. If required, insert the test strip into the meter. Some meters turn on when you insert the strip. Now:

1. Prepare your finger. Holding your hand below your heart, gently milk the finger from the palm to the tip. Prick on the side of the finger, not directly on the top or in the center. The pads of the fingers are very sensitive. The sides have fewer nerves and more blood vessels. A concert pianist with diabetes didn't want to blood test because he was worried it would make his fingers too sore to play. His doctor advised him to do his test on the finger he least used for playing and to use the exact same place every day. That way, a small callus would develop and there would be very little discomfort.

    Arms, palms, and legs can be tested so the fingers don't have to have so many pokes. However, fingertips have the best circulation and other areas show glucose results more slowly. If you are using other areas for blood tests, use them first thing in the morning, before a meal, or at bedtime. Use fingertips for tests performed 1-2 hours after a meal.

2.   Prick your finger. Wipe off the first drop. Milking gently, wait for
      a large blood drop to form. Then turn your finger over and briefly
      touch the drop of blood to the target area on the test strip, covering
      it with blood. Don't touch the strip with your finger. Press a cotton
      ball or tissue to the puncture spot on your finger until the bleeding
      has stopped. If you lick your finger after you test, many people
      with diabetes say their fingertips don't hurt.

3.   Read and record. Read the result and record it in your daily diary,
      even if your meter has a memory.

4.   Discard. Properly discarding your used testing materials is an
      important responsibility. They contain traces of blood and we are all
      much more cautious about blood contaminated wastes these days.
      You can easily wrap your used test strip and cotton ball or tissue in a
      paper towel and throw it in the garbage. The disposal of the used
      lancet and needle portion of your syringe is a different matter. In
      most states the law requires that users of insulin syringes and lancets
      place them in a leak-proof, puncture-resistant container that is closed
      to prevent loss of contents when disposed. Check with your local
      garbage company to find out how to dispose of medical waste in
      your area. To obey the law, do not throw syringe containers in your
      regular garbage. You might be able to purchase a container that
      includes disposal from your pharmacist. When you're away from
      home, break the needle off the end of your syringe (if you're injecting
      insulin) and put it, along with your used lancet, in the carry case for
      your diabetes treasures. You can safely discard it when you get home.

care of your treasures

It's important to properly care for your diabetes supplies. Deborah carries
her supplies in a small, insulated backpack that protects her insulin and
test strips from extreme heat or cold. She keeps her treasures with her at all
times. You can find special carrying cases that have compartments for your

meter, lancets, and test strips, (plus swabs, insulin, and syringes, if you need them.) It's a good idea to also carry extra batteries with you.

Regarding your meter, it's generally a good idea to check the batteries once a week. Also, check your test strips. To be certain that your test strips have not expired, look at the expiration date on the vial before you buy them and when you use them. You can also use manufacturer's directions to check your test strips with a quality-control solution. You should perform a quality-control test every time you open a new vial of strips or whenever your test results do not agree with how you feel. You should also perform it if the vial of strips is left uncapped. Test strips can absorb moisture from the air, affecting their accuracy.

There are times you will experience errors in testing. They can occur when strips that have been exposed to too much heat, cold, or humidity during shipping or while you have had them with you. Tests may be inaccurate if you are extremely anemic. They can also vary with altitude, temperature, and high humidity, and when you have low blood pressure, not enough oxygen in the blood, or high triglycerides. You'll get errors if the strips have expired or you're using the wrong code. Some meters require a chip or strip to calibrate a new bottle of strips; others automatically calibrate.

With some reflectonic-type meters, the blood sample required for the strip may come in contact with the meter and fall over the optic window. You can clean the window by following the manufacturer's directions. If you have any worries about your meter's accuracy, take your meter with you when you have your blood tested at the doctor's office. Perform a test with your meter to compare with the doctor's lab results. They should compare within 15 percent.

oral medications

In the past few years there has been an explosion of new medications to treat Type 2 diabetes. These medications cause a decrease in blood sugar and some also benefit cholesterol levels. The target decrease from each type of medicine is to reduce average blood glucose by 15–60 points. Most people need more than one medication to control their blood glucose.

What are the different classes of oral medications?

+ Biguanide—*Glucophage* is an example of this kind of drug. It reduces insulin resistance and is often associated with weight loss.
+ Alpha glucosidase inhibitors—*Precose* and *Glyset* are taken with meals to slow the breakdown of carbohydrates to simple sugars and prevent high blood sugar after meals.
+ Sulfonylureas—*Amaryl, Glucotrol, Diabeta, Glynase,* and *Diabinese* all stimulate the pancreas to make more insulin. This group is taken once or twice a day.
+ Meglitinides and phenylalanines—*Prandin* and *Starlix* stimulate a brief release of insulin and should be taken with meals to lower your blood sugar after meals.
+ TZDs—*Actos* and *Avandia* are also called glitizones. They increase insulin sensitivity to help it get into the cells.

Combinations of these medications include:

+ *Metaglip*—*Glipizide* and *Metformin* are combined to stimulate the pancreas to produce insulin and to help overcome insulin resistance.
+ *Glucovance*—*Glyburide* and *Metformin* in combination stimulate the pancreas to produce insulin and overcome insulin resistance.
+ *Avandamet*—*Avandia* and *Metformin* combine to overcome insulin resistance and decrease glucose formation in the liver.

Just as this book was nearing completion, Dr. Tim sent me information about some new drugs that involve glucose regulation hormones of the pancreas and stomach. Exenatide, known as *Byetta*, is an incretin, a hormone that was discovered in the saliva of the Gila Monster that provides similar control to long-acting insulin, but causes weight loss rather than weight gain. It is given by injection with the most common side effect being nausea. Amylin is a pancreatic hormone known by the name *Symlyn*, and is given by injection three times daily. It works by slowing stomach emptying and decreasing caloric intake while increasing insulin.

Because exenatide and amylin are injectable, they have limited use. Long-acting injections lasting 1-4 weeks will be available in the future. For patients who want to lose rather than gain weight, these may be a great alternative used alone or with insulin. Since these medications delay gastric emptying, they should be used early in diabetes before any problems with stomach emptying (gastroparesis) occur.

Follow your doctor's directions exactly concerning how and when to take your pills. *Write down a master list of the following:*

✦ The name of your diabetes medicine

✦ How your diabetes medicine works

✦ The exact dose you are to take

✦ What time to take it

✦ When to eat your meals to balance your diabetes medicine

Another new class of medications, the glitizars, marketed as *Pargluva* and *Galida*, have been shown to improve blood glucose levels and to improve blood lipid levels better than the TZD medications. They are otherwise similar to *Actos* and *Avandia*.

Be aware that you can't just pop those pills and then not eat. With diabetes, consistency counts. Eat your meals on time and take your pills as prescribed. It's also important that you know what side effects to watch for. Some diabetes medicines may give you a skin rash or an upset stomach. If this happens, call your doctor or pharmacist immediately. Read all the accompanying literature from your pharmacist and ask questions if you have them.

Be sure to tell your doctor and pharmacist the name of every over-the-counter medication, herb, and natural remedy you take, even aspirin and cough syrup. Sometimes, diabetes drugs do not mix well with other medicines/remedies. If you like wine with dinner or a cocktail at the end of the day, talk with your doctor. Many diabetes medications do not mix well with beer, wine, or liquor.

If, in spite of taking your medication as recommended, your blood sugars are still not in the target range after a few days, don't wait three or four months until your next check-up to tell your doctor or diabetes educator. Call right away. For one thing, using medicines to keep blood sugar at the normal level is not an exact science. It may take quite a bit of trial and error to find what works best for your body. Also, some oral medications may work for a while, and then stop working. If this happens to you, you may need to change medications or take insulin shots.

Please remember that taking pills (or insulin) is not a substitute for taking good care of your body. The pills are relieving a symptom—high blood sugar, but they are not correcting the underlying "dis-ease" process. It's your job to give your body a fighting chance by being at normal body weight, eating healthy foods, and exercising at recommended levels. That way, you reduce your insulin resistance and make it easier to control your blood sugar levels, with or without medication.

There's one more oral medication to add to the list: take a daily multivitamin supplement. In a study reported in the *Annals of Internal Medicine*, March 2003, of 130 people who took a multivitamin for one year, only 17 percent with Type 2 diabetes got the flu or upper respiratory infection, compared with 93 percent who took a placebo.

one pill makes you larger, one pill makes you small

Prescription drugs go through rigorous testing to ensure their safety. Yet despite these regulations, drugs are chemicals and don't always react in predictable ways. When we ingest a drug, it's broken down into molecules that hook up to specific sites called receptors to produce a desired effect, such as lessening pain or lowering blood pressure. Sometimes it takes more than one drug to achieve a desired effect. For example, some people use a diuretic and a blood pressure pill to control their hypertension. Some people have more than one condition, perhaps diabetes and angina, and need a different medication for each.

When the molecules of these drugs interact, two things can happen. First, the drug molecules can hook up to each other instead of the proper receptor site, resulting in an unforeseen reaction. Second, one drug can interfere with the absorption of the other, causing it either not to be absorbed or to be absorbed too rapidly. These processes are referred to as drug interactions. Drug interactions can also occur between over-the-counter (OTC) medications, with drugs and certain foods, and between drugs and the sun.

Jim was a city worker who loved to exercise, but who had pain in his ankles and knees. He started taking glucosamine sulfate to see if that would help his joints. Within a few months, there was marked improvement and he was once again able to bicycle and take long hikes. Then he was diagnosed with Type 2 diabetes. He got his blood sugar under control with diet and exercise, and took Lipitor to lower his cholesterol.

One day Jim felt very dizzy. His blood pressure was 230/120. He was taken to the hospital. Cardiac and neurologic studies were done and he was kept on a heart monitor for days. All his tests were completely normal and during his hospitalization, his symptoms ceased. (He had stopped taking his supplements while he was in the hospital.) At home he restarted his usual routine, including taking supplements, and in a week his symptoms returned. He wasn't even able to drive and missed several days of work. He got a second opinion and was diagnosed with a reaction to glucosamine sulfate. He discontinued using it and his symptoms disappeared.

Glucosamine sulfate is a popular supplement for joint pain. The day after I wrote Jim's story I read an article that described clinical studies that had shown glucosamine sulfate at up to 1500 milligrams a day to be safe for those with diabetes. Yet Dr. Tim's experience with one patient contradicts the research conclusions. Dr. Tim theorizes that some people who take glucosamine sulfate may experience increased uptake of glucose into the nerves that causes the seizures, weakness, and nerve pain.

Drug interactions are more common than one might think and can be serious. A 1989 study found that 9.4 percent of admissions to hospitals were prescription-drug related. Of those, 78 percent occurred in patients over 65 years old. These patients were taking an average of 6.3 medications at the time of their admission.

What can you do to avoid dangerous drug interactions? A long-term relationship with an individual pharmacist is the best insurance against drug interactions. It's his or her job to keep your medication profile, so that all of your medication information is with a single source. Your part in your personal drug-interaction protection plan is to check with your pharmacist every time a new medication is added or when you're going to take an over-the-counter medication. Also, carry a list of your medications with the dosage information in your wallet. If you have more than one doctor, show them the list of all the medications you're taking. If you are concerned about the possibility of a drug interaction, consult your pharmacist or physician immediately.

the greatest treasure of all

Since moving to the mountains six years ago, my husband, René, and I have become involved in an occasional pastime—bird watching. We don't go tromping off into the woods with binoculars. We merely sit on our patio and watch the many bird feeders we've placed around the yard. Recently a Steller's jay honored our patio umbrella with her nest. Steller's jays are bright blue with a black topknot that resembles *Seinfeld*'s Cosmo Kramer's hair. First there was an empty nest, then four spotted blue eggs, then a quartet of scrawny little heads surrounding startled eyes. We've checked on them several times a day and have enjoyed noting their progress.

"They're getting big so quickly!"

"Their topknots are starting to grow!"

"Their wings are turning blue!"

In the last day or so, they've been peering over the side of the nest. My neighbor tells me we'll soon witness the next exciting stage—the first day of flight. They're developing according to their own time line; there's nothing I can do to rush their moment of first flight. Their mother will nudge and when they are ready, they will fly.

Just like the Steller's jay, there are stages we go through, especially when we've been told we have a chronic disease like diabetes. Annalee Shein knows about those stages. She's lived through several of them as the mother of a son who has diabetes. Her son was fourteen when he was diagnosed and his first reactions are familiar to us all: anger, denial, and fear. Annalee knew about diabetes and what it can do if you don't take care of it: her father died from diabetic complications.

She told me, "My son went through several difficult years, so difficult that, at times, I feared for his life. As I learned how to give him the love and support that got him through that time, I realized that I had something to give to others."

When her son went off to college, so did she. She got her bachelor's degree in psychology in 1991, her Master's in Social Work in 1993, and became a certified social worker. Working with adolescents and their families, she's developed a tool she calls the "Four A's," the stages of living with diabetes. They are:

awareness

This is the first step. You can't deal with something if you're not aware of it. This may sound obvious, yet we know there are many, many people in our country who have diabetes and don't know it until they begin to have eye problems or nerve damage. The awareness stage is often accompanied by strong emotions. "It's not fair. Why did I have to get diabetes? What did I do wrong?" You may feel cheated, betrayed. Diabetes directly confronts the illusion that you're in control. You may want to blame someone or something, an ancestor or relative or God, for "giving" you diabetes.

Annalee notes, "This is a big issue for teenagers. They think they're invincible. Then a teen gets diabetes. He understands that his life is now in his own hands. Teens face their mortality. It's almost as if they go through a midlife crisis as a teen. It's a real slap in the face."

I think diabetes is a slap in the face for anyone. It's even more difficult if you haven't been paying much attention to your health, because you're going to be asked to make drastic changes in your lifestyle. You'll need to become aware of what you eat, when you eat, and how it affects your blood sugar, plus the discipline of daily blood tests and medication.

✦ ✦ ✦

acknowledgment

This is the stage of beginning to care for yourself. A few of us make a quick decision to learn it all and get it really right (mostly the control freaks among us). Some of us balk at the idea of so much daily discipline. For some of us, it's a bit-by-bit venture. "Okay, I've got diabetes. I'll take my pills or my shots. But don't bother me with all this diet and blood testing. That's too much to ask. I'll be fine." That might do for a little while, but if that approach continues for very long, it will lead to serious problems. Whatever your perspective, trying to make so many changes at once can be overwhelming.

Acknowledgment is a vital step toward living successfully with diabetes. It's admitting, "It's here and it won't go away." This stage can take some time. You may find yourself fighting this step, wishing it would just go away. You may feel as if pushing it away somehow makes it less real. If "wishing and hoping and thinking and praying" could make it so, Brennan would have parted ways with diabetes a long time ago.

Sometimes this stage of acknowledgment is accompanied by the mind spewing out despairing thoughts of how you're now less than you were, you're damaged, and your life is ruined by this something that's "wrong" with you. A quick word about that kind of thinking: stop it as quickly as you can. I remember going through the same thoughts about my son. I had been so proud of his good health, but now "something was wrong with him." I caught myself thinking this as Brennan came through the room, laughing and chasing his brother. I suddenly realized that my son was the same child he had always been. I was accepting the idea that people with disabilities or diseases were different, less "perfect" than the rest of us. What nonsense! Brennan was a perfectly normal little boy. He just had a pancreas that wasn't working as well as it should.

The same is true for you. Even though you've got diabetes, you are the same "you" you've always been. Your body is having a problem and it's your job to pay attention to its cries for help. That's all that's happened. All the most interesting parts of you—the love you have to give, the care, the wisdom, the talents and the flaws—all of it is still there to be used for life's great journey. If you don't believe me, bring to mind someone like Christopher Reeve. People who overcome challenges become known as heroes. Maybe life is asking you to be a hero—to your children, to your parents, to your friends, and to other people with diabetes. Nothing stands in your way of meeting this challenge except the thoughts you have about your abilities and your situation.

At the same time, there may be sadness in this part of the process. You had expectations, even if you'd never clearly stated them, and I'm sure they didn't include diabetes. But it's here now and you have to decide what you're going to do about it. The challenge of diabetes is going to ask you to grow and change and learn. As writer Rita Mae Brown says, "People are like tea bags. You never know how strong they'll be until they're in hot water."

acceptance

This is a major step forward. You embrace (yes, I did say embrace) diabetes as a new life companion. You conclude as Nicole Johnson, Miss America 1999 did, "I'm the one who's responsible for my diabetes. No one else can do it for me."

For many adults, acceptance can be a tough challenge. Sometimes we feel that having diabetes means we'll be deprived of the things we worked for which we now deserve to enjoy. Yet I assure you that you can have a happy and productive life while balancing the demands of diabetes.

What will help you get to acceptance? Dr. Tim treats a number of children with Type 2 who are in their teens. He's observed that there isn't one specific teaching that brings any of them to acceptance. He says, "We find the shift occurs at a different point for each person. It usually involves a sudden realization, 'Oh, this is my problem, not my parents', and I can do something about it.' Then they begin to exercise and eat properly, and everything changes. They have success and their self-image improves. Very few get their weight back to normal, but some lose thirty to forty pounds. They look and feel better. They have to buy new clothes. Their friends comment on the improvement and that encourages them to keep up the effort."

Acceptance can lead to transformation. A patient named Ann recently told Dr. Tim, "Diabetes is the best thing that's ever happened to me in my life. I've lost weight, I wear the clothes I love, my blood pressure and cholesterol are fine, and I have lots of energy again. Everybody has noticed the change in me and they're asking me what I'm doing." What she's doing is finally taking really good care of herself!

action

You're ready to take the tools you've been given to control diabetes and put them to work. You do it because it's the way you can take back a measure of control. You can't control everything that happens to you, but you can control how you respond to what life brings your way. You find yourself saying things like, "I'm going to make sure I get to the doctor on schedule. I'm going to pay attention to my food intake. I'm going to get the right amount of exercise. I'm okay the way I am—with diabetes. My life is worth the effort it will take to keep me healthy."

So, which stage are you in? If you've haven't made your way to the fourth stage, do you have any thoughts about what will help you get there?

one more a

All these A's add up to the most important A of all, eh? (That's for my Canadian friends.) Attitude. For inspiration in this department, we turn our hymnals to the Clayton Harmon page.

Clayton was diagnosed with diabetes in November 1950. He recalls, "My doctor's name was Woodard E. Farmer. I looked on him as one of the best doctors who came down the pike. He diagnosed me right quickly, handed me a book from the Joslin Clinic, and said 'You make this your second Bible. You read everything you can about diabetes, because you have to be your own doctor.' That was the best advice I ever had."

Back then Clayton only took one shot a day, a regimen he continued for forty years, until he began having trouble with his eyes. "My eyes went blurry and I went to the eye doctor. He said, 'Have you taken that course over at the hospital?' and I told him no. He recommended it, so I took the course. They put me on four shots a day and I said 'how about three?' But

I saw right away that four was the best. Through the years, there's always been more to learn."

Clayton's a man who knows the value of trying harder. He's seen what diabetes can do. One brother, an uncle, and a cousin all had it and suffered its complications. He told me, "I tell my wife every day that I believe if it weren't for her, I wouldn't be alive today. I was the seventh of eight boys born to my mother September 29th, 1919. All of them are gone now. My last brother died ten years ago. Here I am, still living, despite the fact that I've had diabetes for fifty-one years."

Five years ago, Clayton helped start a support group at the diabetes center. He suggested they call it "the Cornerstone Support Group," based on his belief that each of us is the cornerstone of our own care. Clayton also makes hospital visits to other patients with diabetes. "When I go to visit them, I see every conceivable problem that arises from having diabetes. I make it a point of telling them, 'Look, when you walk out this door, who is responsible for your health? The doctor can only spend so many minutes with you. Then you're on your own; it's up to you.'"

Clayton Harmon knows that his experience of diabetes is in his own hands. He says he loves the phrase, "Your attitude determines your altitude." "I've always been fascinated by the meaning of words," he said. "Whenever I'd hear a word I didn't know, I'd look it up in the dictionary. 'Attitude' is the most important one of all!"

He also knows it's important to have heroes. One of his is Norman Vincent Peale, who wrote *The Power of Positive Thinking*. Another hero of Clayton's is W. Clement Stone, a man well known for promoting "PMA"—Positive Mental Attitude.

If you think you need more than just positive attitude, Clayton has another idea. He remembers what he did fifty-one years ago when he was diagnosed. He prayed. "Lord, you know I have this diabetes, and if you'll go with me, everything will be all right," Clayton adds, "And if anyone is afraid about having diabetes, they should read Psalm 46."

What are your sources of support for living with diabetes? Your primary support comes from the way you think and talk about your diabetes. It is called your "inner dialogue" and it determines your attitude.

And don't forget laughter. *Diabetes Care* reported a study showing the connection between laughter and lower blood glucose levels. Keiko Hayashi, Ph.D., R.N., and his team of researchers at the University of Tsukuba in Ibaraki, Japan, measured the blood glucose levels of twenty-four people—nineteen with Type 2 diabetes and five without—on two separate days before and after they ate the same meal. Immediately following their meal, the patients watched either a forty-minute lecture on a dry topic or a forty-minute comedy show. While blood sugar levels rose in all participants after each meal, the patients who watched the comedy show experienced a significantly smaller increase in blood sugar level than those who watched the lecture did. Laughter is good medicine. Research has shown that laughter can increase your tolerance to pain, lower your risk of heart attack, reduce your levels of stress hormones, and boost your immune system.

Diabetes occasionally provides a laugh. In seventh grade, Brennan came home every day on the school bus. One of the other boys on the bus had auditory dyslexia. Sometimes on the way home, Brennan would begin to feel he had low blood sugar and he'd tell Annie, the bus driver, because she always carried LifeSavers. One afternoon, he was at the back of the bus and yelled, "Annie, send back some LifeSavers. I'm having a reaction!"

When the bus reached Brennan's stop, he got off, followed by the boy with dyslexia who turned to Annie and asked, "Why do you give Brennan LifeSavers when he has an erection?"

I've learned that there are gifts to be found in even the steepest challenges. After thirty-three years of living with diabetes, Larry has found that, for him, diabetes has been a blessing. He says, "It's asked me to pay close attention to my body and my emotions. I think I'm in better overall health because of living so consciously, and I'm more aware of how precious life is."

"Yesterday I was diagnosed with diabetes. Today I need to know ten thousand new things!"

chapter five

everything is upside down

It was the summer of 1980 and Brennan had had diabetes for almost a year. I arrived home shortly after dinner and as I opened the back door, I heard Brennan whining. I found him in his father's office, sitting on the couch, looking miserable. His dad explained that Brennan had been really cranky for the last hour or so. I asked if maybe Brennan had low blood sugar. Alan said he was sure that wasn't it, because Brennan had taken his insulin shot and eaten all his dinner more than forty minutes ago. (This was back in the days when we did urine testing, so we had no way of knowing his exact blood sugar.) To my eye, Brennan was acting exactly as if he were having an insulin reaction. I trusted my instincts and gave Brennan some juice. In a few minutes, the whining stopped and Brennan was his cheerful self again.

Brennan's blood sugar must have been low before he got his insulin injection and the extra insulin brought his blood sugar even lower. He'd eaten enough dinner to keep from passing out or having convulsions, but he was having a prolonged insulin reaction and his brain was not receiving enough fuel.

I asked Brennan if he remembered eating dinner. He didn't. I asked him how he felt. He said, "Mommy, everything was upside down."

Diabetes does seem to turn everything upside down. Normally, blood sugar control is a perfect example of supply and demand. A person eats and the food is broken down into glucose. The pancreas responds to the amount of food eaten by releasing enough insulin to allow the glucose to enter the cells as fuel. With diabetes, the body is not responding adequately to the body's need for insulin, so medication is taken and balanced with a consistent eating plan.

the diabetes teeter-totter

When I was a little girl, I loved to play on the teeter-totter (also known as the seesaw.) Sometimes, I would stand on top, straddling the center support. I'd teeter from side to side, trying to find my balance. At first the board would bang down on one side, then the other. I'd close my eyes, concentrate, and gradually feel the subtleties of reconciling the weight and length of the board. Then the moment came: the board was perfectly parallel to the ground. I'd hold it there, triumphant, then I'd feel it start to move. One end would dip down. I'd shift my weight and bring it up. The other end would dip and I'd shift. It was a game I played by myself, for myself.

Diabetes is a lot like that game I played so many years ago. Balance is achieved when your blood sugar is in the 80 to 120 mg/dl range. Food, medication, and exercise provide leverage. There will be times of balance, but they won't last very long. Your blood sugar will teeter this way and that, above or below your goal. As time goes by, you will discover the subtleties of consistency. It will be a game you play mostly by yourself, for yourself.

Diabetes is one of mankind's oldest diseases, but exactly what caused it wasn't known until 1921 when Dr. Frederick Banting and his medical assistant, Charles Best, discovered insulin. Late in the 1800s, scientists realized that there was a connection between diabetes, "the sugar disease," and the Islets of Langerhans in the pancreas. While reading a paper on the subject, Dr. Banting realized that the digestive juices of the pancreas were destroying its own hormone. He talked his department head at the University of Toronto, John J. R. Macleod, into giving him lab space, a medical assistant and ten dogs. Within a few months, they had conclusive results: when they gave the substance they extracted from the islets of Langerhans (called insulin from the Latin for "island") to diabetic dogs, their high blood sugars were definitively lowered. Within a few months, the insulin search team had isolated enough insulin to give to a fourteen-year-old boy dying of diabetes. His blood sugar plunged and his urine cleared of sugar. Banting and Best published a paper on their discovery in 1922. Banting was awarded the Nobel Prize in 1923, an honor he shared with John Macleod.

The discovery of insulin was a revolutionary moment in medicine. Because of the work of Dr. Banting and Charles Best, Eli Lilly produced the first commercially available insulin using cows and pigs as the source in 1923. Before that year, people diagnosed with diabetes usually lived less than two years. The choice between two years to live and a lifetime of insulin injections seemed like an obvious one to the people who had diabetes at that time. It still is.

insulin therapy

Perhaps the idea of injections is new to you. Dr. Tim has noticed that when a patient is diagnosed with Type 2, one of the first questions is "Do I need insulin?" His answer is always, "Yes, you do need insulin, but not everyone with Type 2 needs insulin injections."

Many people with Type 2 manage it with a combination of meal planning, exercise and oral medications, but, eventually, this approach may not be sufficient. Drugs are limited in how much they can overcome insulin deficiency and resistance. Forty percent of those with Type 2 need injected insulin at some time. It may be because oral medications fail, during hospitalizations, or during times of increased stress. A need for insulin often follows pancreatitis, an inflammation of the pancreas that occurs with high triglycerides, and after trauma or infection.

It's a common misconception among new users of injected insulin that taking more shots is not a good thing. *Diabetes Care* magazine reported that Canadian diabetic patients who are new users of insulin say that reducing the number of injections from twice to once per day is as important as improving glucose control. Not true! Whether it takes one, two, three or even four shots, a successful insulin therapy program brings your blood sugar into the "good control" range as frequently as possible. The purpose of injecting insulin is to mimic, as closely as possible, the body's natural response to eating and the body delivers insulin all day long.

There are two ways the body uses insulin to keep blood sugar in the normal range: the basal rate and the insulin response. In a non-diabetic person, the body always has a small amount of insulin, known as the "basal rate," circulating in the blood. When food is eaten, the pancreas releases more insulin, known as the "insulin response." You'll be approximating the basal rate and the insulin response with the insulin schedule you'll be using.

The amount of insulin needed varies from person to person. Too little or too much insulin can cause problems both great and small. Insulin allows glucose to enter the cells to produce energy. If there's too little insulin, you won't have the energy you need. The body then searches for an energy source, breaking down fat and muscle to try to meet its needs. You begin to lose weight, as my son did, and your body chemistry goes awry. Too much insulin has a different effect. Since insulin is adipogenic (promotes the storage of fat), the more insulin you take or produce, the more weight you gain. Fat increases the body's resistance to insulin, and increases the need for insulin. It's a good example of a vicious cycle.

Your insulin therapy goal is to take just enough insulin for your energy and metabolic needs. Too much and you'll have difficulty with low blood sugar, plus you'll gain weight, which can interfere with your body's balance and put you at risk for additional serious health problems. Too little and you won't have the energy you need for even simple daily tasks, plus your blood sugar will be above target range which is the cause of complications. It's quite a balancing act.

Some people might only need one shot of intermediate-acting insulin at breakfast or at bedtime, possibly combined with oral medication. Others might need short- and intermediate-acting insulin before breakfast and add another injection at dinner. Almost any combination might be recommended.

There are two basic approaches to the use of insulin. One is called "conventional" diabetes therapy. It usually involves two to three shots a day using NPH with Regular, blood testing and following a meal plan. The idea is that the morning dose of NPH or Lente would last during the day and the second dose covers the night. Sometimes an additional shot of NPH is added at bedtime. The morning Regular lasts six to eight hours and covers the meals at breakfast and lunch. The evening Regular covers dinner and a bedtime snack. The doses of insulin generally remain the same each day. It requires that you plan your insulin according to what you think your needs will be for the next six to twelve hours. To use this therapy, you need to be a person who keeps regular hours and has predictable activities. This approach gives adequate, but not optimal, blood sugar control.

We now know it's best to use a physiologic approach to insulin therapy, meaning an approach that replicates the body's own strategies for controlling blood sugar. Research has shown that this kind of intensive therapy results in far fewer complications. This physiologic approach is called "intensive" insulin therapy. It's based on the assumption that your daily activity, eating patterns and metabolism change from day to day. The intensive approach comes closest to replicating your body's natural mechanisms—knowing the current blood sugar level and then providing the right amount of insulin. It also gives you the most flexibility and freedom.

To accomplish intensive therapy, you use one kind of insulin that mimics the basal rate, preferably one that lasts for at least twenty-four hours without peaking. Then you mimic the body's insulin response by taking a shot of fast-acting insulin that lasts three to four hours to cover each meal. For example, if your lunch meeting is delayed by one hour and you're on conventional therapy, you run the risk of the Regular you took in the morning being at its maximum effectiveness when there's no meal to eat. You could easily have a huge drop in blood sugar. With intensive therapy, a delayed lunch is not a problem, because your breakfast fast-acting insulin has diminished in effectiveness by lunchtime. The long-acting is covering your basic needs until your lunch is ready. Then you take your next shot to cover that specific meal.

The ironic part of this is that many people turn to intensive therapy because of erratic blood sugars and higher than recommended HbA1c numbers, yet because this therapy keeps you in the normal range more of the time, you are closer to a low blood sugar reaction. It has been noted that those on intensive therapy have more frequent low blood sugar episodes. With intensive therapy, you keep yourself in the normal range to avoid long-term complications, but to do so successfully, you must pay consistent attention to the details of control or risk frequent insulin reactions.

If diabetes is new to you, you may be put on conventional therapy while learning the basics of insulin use. If after a reasonable period of time your HbA1c readings aren't at or below 6.5, talk with your doctor about using intensive insulin therapy.

To understand the difference in the two types of insulin therapy, look at Figure 1. It shows you how blood sugar rises after meals.

Figure 1—Glucose Rise After Meals and Snacks

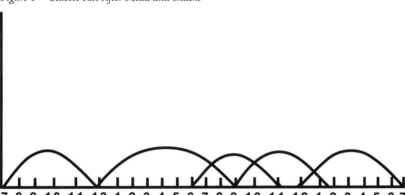

Now look at Figure 2. You'll see how Regular and NPH given in two injections a day covers the rise in blood sugar after meals. Notice how the effectiveness peaks and then diminishes.

Figure 2—Two Injections of Regular and NPH

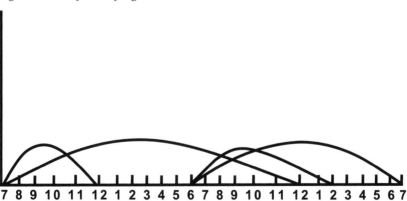

Look at the combination of long-acting Lantus with fast-acting Humalog or Novolog. Do you see how much more closely it mimics the pattern of blood sugar rise shown in Figure 1?

Long-acting Lantus or Levemir insulin

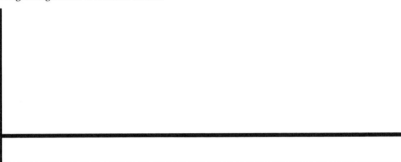

Long-acting Lantus or Levemir with Humalog or Novolog before meals

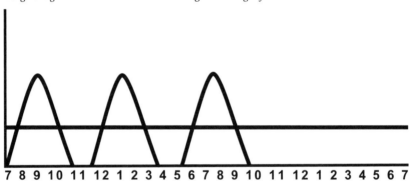

NPH intermediate-acting twice daily with short acting regular insulin

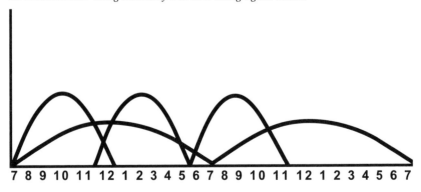

These illustrations clearly show that the newer insulins offer improved blood sugar control.

syringes, pumps, and pens

There are currently two ways to get insulin into your body—through individual injections or by insulin infusion pump. The syringe is the most widely used delivery method in the U.S. By the way, you can safely reuse your syringes. If the needle has only touched your skin and the insulin bottle, you can reuse it several times until it is dull. Just carefully recap it after each use. Many people do this because the cost of diabetes supplies is so high. One exception: Lantus is made up of long crystals that clog the needle tip and a syringe for Lantus should only be used once.

The insulin pump is one of the great advances in diabetes care. It's worn on the outside of the body and delivers insulin by way of tubing connected to a needle that stays in place for several days at a time. Pumps use buffered Regular, Humalog, or Novalog insulin, releasing a slow, steady flow that mimics the way the pancreas naturally provides the basal insulin supply. Then the user releases additional insulin at meals, known as a bolus. The bolus replicates the "insulin response." Researchers haven't figured out quite yet how to make an inner blood sugar sensor that would make the insulin pump a self-correcting machine, so it's important for pump users to test their blood sugar frequently.

Compared to a syringe, an insulin pump is a complex system, but it does come closest to mimicking normal insulin release. For some people, use of the pump can result in blood sugars very close to target range when other strategies have failed. A pump is not a cure: It doesn't allow you to abandon the elements of good diabetes control—meal planning, exercise, and blood testing. Many doctors recommend trying intensive insulin therapy with three or four injections a day to achieve control before moving to the expense and complexity of a pump. If you and your doctor decide the pump is for you, you will be given special instruction and guidance, plus the manufacturer will provide an 800 number you can call for additional information.

In the U.S., 95 percent of people with diabetes use syringes to inject insulin, but in Europe, 95 percent use insulin pens with ultra fine needles. Insulin pens offer a discreet way to use insulin. They are the same size and shape as a fountain pen and easily fit in your pocket or purse. Some people like pens because they don't have to load insulin from bottles: the insulin can be dialed up from a cartridge. The drawback of using a pen is its higher cost, plus the fact that you can only use one kind of insulin at a time unless you're using premixed insulin of NPH and Regular. Your educator can advise you about using pens and premixed insulin.

If you're using a disposable insulin pen, first tip the pen back and forth twenty times to gently mix the contents. Then attach the needle and proceed. For non-disposable pens, drop the insulin cartridge into the pen, put the top back on, and shake the pen back and forth twenty times to mix. Follow the instructions that come with your particular pen to remove air bubbles. Dial the dose of insulin you need. If you are using two types of insulin, you will need to have two insulin pens and give yourself two injections.

Most people like to perform their shots in private, but some people give injections through their clothes when they're in public. I have a friend who does that and I read that a researcher at Wayne State University School of Medicine studied this approach and found it was both convenient and safe.

For many years, researchers have been working on new insulin delivery systems. One has finally arrived: inhaled insulin. Since the air sacks of the lung have as large a surface area as a tennis court, this has seemed like a good place to put insulin into the body. Four new types of inhaled insulin systems have been developed, but currently the FDA has only approved Exubera. It's comparable to short-acting insulin. It begins working within fifteen minutes and may last up to five hours, so often only two doses are needed, for breakfast and for the evening meal. Inhaled insulin will be especially helpful for people who refuse injections because of the fear of shots, more finger pokes for blood testing, fear of hypoglycemia, and worry about weight gain. Exubera solves the fear of shots problem and also has been shown to have less hypoglycemia associated with it. One side effect has been observed: 30% of patients experience some coughing. Also for those with asthma, the absorption rate varies.

kinds of insulin

There are four basic kinds of insulin: rapid, short, intermediate, and long-acting. Each type varies according to how quickly it begins to work, (onset); when it works the hardest, (peak activity); and how long it works, (duration).

Rapid-acting begins to work within fifteen minutes and lasts from three to five hours. Humalog and Novolog fit in this category. They should be given 1–15 minutes before a meal.

Short-acting Regular lasts up to eight hours and should be given thirty minutes before a meal. There's also buffered Regular insulin, a special insulin used in insulin pumps.

Intermediate-acting NPH and Lente begin to work within 1 1/2 hours and last from fourteen to sixteen hours.

There are also Lantus and Levemir, which begin to work within 1 1/2 hours, last for up to 24 hours, and do not peak, which helps lessen the chance of insulin reactions. Lantus has other advantages over the other long-acting insulins. Because it doesn't peak, it's less likely to cause low blood sugar at night and is associated with less weight gain.

Lantus does require special handling. It cannot be mixed with other insulins and must be injected from a separate syringe. It's usually given at bedtime, but I recently heard from a friend who switched her Lantus injection to the morning. She was having trouble with very low morning blood sugar—in the 40s range. She and her doctor believe that because she wasn't eating during those sleep hours, the action of the Lantus was a little too vigorous for her. She takes Lantus in the morning and its action is winding down while she's sleeping. Her before-breakfast blood sugar, twenty-four hours after she takes the Lantus, is in the 120 to 140 range. She and her doctor are now working on getting that down a little closer to 80. (I tell you this story to let you know that sometimes you and your doctor can get creative. Not everyone reacts the same way to a particular insulin. What works for one person may not work for another. Your job is to work with your doctor to find an approach that is effective for you.)

One more thing about Lantus: Three people I know who recently switched to Lantus are extremely happy they did, but the switch-over was difficult. It took them more than one month for their bodies to adjust. During the adjustment period, their blood sugars were erratic and it was very frustrating. Knowing ahead of time that the adjustment period was going to be extended helped the process. As one friend said, "I'm glad another friend with diabetes told me that my switching to Lantus could cause my body to react so unpredictably at first. It helped me be more patient. I took several weeks to settle down, but now my blood sugars are better than ever."

There's a newer long-acting insulin, similar to Lantus, that has recently come on the market. It's called Levimir, is given once or twice daily and, just like Lantus, cannot be mixed in the same syringe with other insulins.

There are also pre-mixed insulins which combine rapid or short-acting with intermediate-acting, so that you don't have to load two insulins into one syringe. These can be helpful for some people. They come in several strengths and combinations. You can discuss their use with your doctor or educator.

buying and caring for insulin

When you buy insulin, check the insulin box and label carefully. Make sure you get the exact insulin your doctor wants you to take. Using the wrong insulin can greatly affect your diabetes control. You need to know these facts about your insulin in order to buy the right kind:

- ♦ Brand Name: Nova Nordisk, Eli Lilly, Aventis
- ♦ Type: NPH, Regular, Lente, Novolog, Humalog, Lantus, Levemir
- ♦ Concentration: U-100 or U-40. U-100 is primarily used in the U.S.
- ♦ Expiration Date

Insulin is measured in units. A unit is a small amount of pure insulin. Most bottles of insulin sold in the United States have 100 units of insulin in each milliliter of fluid. This is called U-100 insulin. The amount of insulin in a milliliter is its concentration. There are two concentrations: U-100 and

U-40. In countries outside the United States, U-40 insulin is in common use and there is a small amount of U-40 insulin sold in the United States. Since most insulin bottles hold 10 milliliters of fluid, a bottle of U-100 insulin contains 1000 units.

The syringes you buy must match the concentration of your insulin. If you use U-100 insulin, your syringes should have orange tops and say U-100 on the package. Syringes come in 30 unit, 50 unit, and 100 unit sizes. With needles, the higher the number indicated the smaller the needle's diameter. You can use 29 or 30 gauge needles. Some ultra-fine needles come in 31 gauge, not much larger than a human hair.

How long will a bottle of insulin last? Check the expiration date on the insulin box before you buy it. The date printed on the box must allow enough time for you to use the whole bottle. To find out how long the bottle needs to last, divide the number of units in the bottle by the number of units you take each day. (Remember each 10 milliliter bottle of U-100 insulin contains 1000 units.)

Example 1: 1000 units U-100 NPH divided by 35 units per day = 28 days. In this case, if you start a new bottle of NPH on March 1, you will finish it on March 28. You should not buy a bottle with an expiration date earlier than March 28.

Example 2: 1000 units of U-100 R divided by 15 units per day = 66 days. In this case, if you start a new bottle of regular insulin on March 1, you will finish it on May 5. You should not buy a bottle with an expiration date earlier than May 5.

Warning note: All of the new insulins—Lantus, Humalog, and Novalog—should be discarded twenty-eight days following the first injection from that vial. Some Lantus users have noticed that its effectiveness lasts less than 28 days from the day they opened the bottle. They find themselves having higher blood sugars after using a bottle of Lantus for twenty-two or twenty-three days. They also find it frustrating to pay for insulin they then have to throw away! You can discuss this with your doctor or diabetes educator.

Always keep an extra bottle of insulin or box of insulin cartridges on hand. When you begin using your last bottle, buy another immediately.

✦ ✦ ✦

storing insulin

Insulin is a protein and temperature extremes can lessen its effectiveness. The bottle or cartridge of insulin you are currently using can be kept at room temperature, but don't let it get too warm or too cold. There are special carriers made for traveling with insulin supplies, but something as simple as a thermos container can be used. (Ask your doctor or diabetes educator, or go online to www. medicool.com to view a variety of insulated and non-insulated carrying cases for your diabetes supplies.) Keep your unrefrigerated insulin out of direct sunlight. Don't leave it in the car unless it's being kept cool in an insulated bag. If the temperature in your house is above 80 degrees, keep your insulin in the refrigerator, but never let it freeze.

Keep extra insulin in a warmer part of the refrigerator, like the butter compartment. If you need to use a new bottle that's been chilled, you can warm it up before injecting it. Fill the syringe and hold it between your palms until it reaches room temperature.

Treat your insulin gently. Don't shake it vigorously. Don't let it get tossed around. Insulin that is handled roughly is more likely to clump or frost. To mix it before use, gently roll the bottle between your hands or tilt cartridges back and forth twenty times.

If you're concerned that your insulin may no longer be usable, check its color and clarity. Lantus, Humalog, Novalog Regular, and Buffered Regular insulins should be clear and have no color. Do not use any of these if they look cloudy, thickened, slightly colored, or if they have any solid particles in them.

Semilente, NPH, Lente, premixed 70/30 and 50/50, Ultralente, and PZI insulins should have an even, cloudy appearance similar to skim milk. If there are clumps of insulin in the liquid or on the bottom after shaking or if solid particles of insulin stick to the bottom or sides of the bottle after gentle shaking, making the bottle look frosted on the inside, don't use them.

✦ ✦ ✦

injections

Seventy-two-year-old Kathy had had Type 2 diabetes for three years. During a physical examination, Dr. Tim noticed she'd lost some sensation in her feet due to diabetic neuropathy. Kathy had been taking oral medications, but her HbA1c was still 8.0, meaning she had an average blood glucose of 180. When Dr. Tim suggested it was time to begin insulin injections, she replied, "You can't make me take insulin."

Dr. Tim agreed. He knew he couldn't "make" her take insulin. He asked if he could give her an injection of saline (salt water) using an insulin syringe as an experiment. She agreed. Using an ultra-fine needle, he painlessly injected the salt water. Kathy was stunned. She thought injections had to be painful. She began using preloaded Novalog 70/30 insulin and after four months, her hemoglobin A1c was down to 6.7.

The idea of piercing one's skin with a needle every day isn't pleasurable. Thinking about giving injections over the weeks, months, and years ahead may seem like an impossible task. The good news is that you only have to take one injection at a time. When Brennan was diagnosed, I remember being shown a line drawing of a child's body with small dots lined up across the upper arms, thighs, and stomach. These were all the places I would stick my child with needles. I almost fainted. Yet Brennan was concerned with only one injection: the one happening at that moment. He didn't look ahead or fuss about an injection he'd be taking later that day.

If your mind starts to conjure a despairing picture of syringes, bottles, and other paraphernalia, stop for a moment and take a breath. Let go of the future and practice what is called "child's mind." Children live in the moment. They don't project what will be. They see what is. Remind yourself there's only one shot to be concerned with—the one you're taking right now. Just as you can't live or breathe in the future, you will never take a future injection, only the one right here, right now, the one that will be over in just a few moments.

There's much you can do to help injections be more comfortable. The discomfort of shots comes from two things: the needle going through the skin and the spreading of the tissues by the fluid that's being injected. Use the thinnest, sharpest needle you can buy and insert it quickly. Take a deep breath through your nose and blow through pursed lips, like blowing out a candle, just as you insert the needle. Also, don't inject cold insulin. As mentioned, keep your current bottle at room temperature.

The atmosphere at shot time is important. If you've been rushing, take a few deep breaths in and out through your nose to calm yourself. You might take a moment to imagine the way the insulin is helping your body stay healthy and balanced. In spite of how you may initially feel about taking shots, for you insulin is a blessing. Without it you would not be around for very long to enjoy your friends and family. There are countries where children and adults do not have adequate access to insulin. You do. Gratitude is appropriate.

choosing the injection site

The white areas in the two drawings shown indicate where injections can be given, although you may need assistance to reach some of those pictured. In the illustrations, the areas are divided into squares. To keep skin, fat, and muscle healthy, it is important to use a different site for each shot.

Give insulin injections into the white areas on a rotating basis.

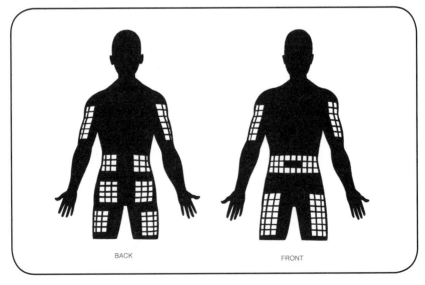

BACK   FRONT

Your diabetes educator will recommend which sites you should begin using. Over the weeks and months ahead, you'll notice how your body responds to insulin injected at those sites. Since the goal is to have consistent blood sugar readings, you may find that using certain sites will help you achieve that.

For over ten years, Susan has given her injections solely in her abdomen. Her endocrinologist told her that insulin would act more consistently if she gave all her injections in her stomach. The reason is that by injecting in the stomach you run less risk of the insulin being slowed by the larger muscles in the legs, arms, or bottom. Except for Deborah's bottom, left one to be exact. Deborah and her mother learned many years ago that injecting into her left hip would cause her blood sugar to drop very quickly. Her mom called it the "bear-watching bottom." Her mom knew that if Deborah had her morning shot in that hip, her blood sugar that day would "bear watching," because the insulin would absorb so quickly that there was a strong tendency she'd have a low blood sugar episode.

Jeffrey, a computer programmer, had the opposite problem. During one project, Jeffrey was working twelve to fourteen hours a day and snacking out of vending machines. He didn't have insurance and didn't want to use too many of his glucose testing strips, so he tried to guess the amount of insulin he needed. After a few days, he found he couldn't concentrate or make decisions, so he tested his blood sugar. Initially it was in the 200s, then the 300s, and then almost 500. He thought his insulin had stopped working, so he purchased new insulin, but it didn't bring his blood sugars down.

Jeffrey had been giving his insulin in exactly the same place every day. He was right-handed, so he gave the insulin in the left side of his abdomen. All the injections were within an inch of each other and he had developed scar tissue in the region. The scar tissue had resulted in poor insulin absorption. He started to rotate his insulin injection sites and within a few days, his blood sugars were once again controlled.

Your diabetes educator will advise you about site rotation: following a regular pattern as you move your shots from site to site. Keeping track of your rotation pattern will help you remember where to give your next shot. Site rotation is used because each time you inject insulin, it breaks down the underlying tissue a little and, if that site is used too frequently, as we read in Jeffrey's case, scar tissue forms. It's usually advisable to use all the sites in one area before changing to another. For example, you might use all the sites in both arms before moving to your legs. If you take more than one shot each day, you may use a different area for each shot, perhaps using the abdomen in the morning and your legs at night when you're less active.

Different people use different patterns. You might start in a corner of an area, then move down or across the injection sites in order. Jumping from site to site makes it hard to remember where you gave your last shot. When you have used all the sites in an area, you can start over in that area or move to another.

It's also good for you to know your body's absorption rate from these different areas. There may be times you choose to use an area because of how quickly or slowly insulin is taken up. If you'll be eating very soon after a shot, you might use a site on your stomach as it absorbs rather quickly. If you use a hot tub, you wouldn't want to inject insulin prior to bathing because heat encourages insulin to be absorbed faster and drop your blood sugar more quickly.

injecting two types of insulin

Your diabetes educator will teach you this process, but here it is again—a quick tutorial. Unless you are using commercial premixed insulin, load your syringe just before your shot. If you premix two insulins in a syringe and store them for future use, you will end up with erratic absorption of insulin as some of the insulin will bind to the syringe walls. Also, when some insulins are mixed, they can begin to interact chemically after only ten minutes.

Parts of a syringe

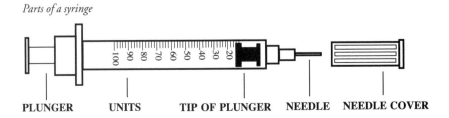

PLUNGER   UNITS   TIP OF PLUNGER   NEEDLE   NEEDLE COVER

Note: If you're using only one insulin, skip step #3, except for tapping the air bubbles out of the syringe.

1.   Mix. Gently roll the bottle of long-acting insulin between your hands to mix it; do not shake it. Medical personnel may tell you to wipe the top of the bottle with an alcohol swab. I stopped using alcohol swabs early on as the alcohol irritated Brennan's skin. Dr. Tim says it's not really necessary if you keep your insulin in a clean place. Discuss the use of alcohol swabs with your educator or doctor.

2.   Inject air into the first bottle. Pull the plunger to the desired number of units of your long-acting insulin to fill the bottle with that amount of air. Holding the bottle upside down, inject the air into the center of the bottle. Putting air in makes it easier to draw insulin out. Withdraw the syringe.

3.   Inject air into the second bottle and withdraw insulin. Now repeat the process with the bottle of short-acting insulin: drawing the desired units of air into the syringe and injecting the air into that bottle. Keeping that bottle upside down, pull the plunger out slowly, drawing the insulin into the syringe until you get the exact number of units needed. Withdraw the syringe from the bottle. Remove any air bubbles by tapping the syringe with your finger. Air bubbles are not dangerous when injected into fatty tissue or muscle, but they do take up space in the syringe that should be taken by insulin. More air bubbles, less insulin.

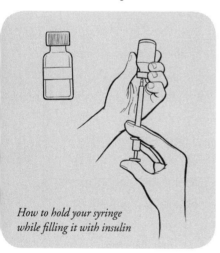

How to hold your syringe while filling it with insulin

4.   Withdraw insulin from first bottle. Insert the syringe in the bottle of long-acting, holding it upside down and pull the plunger out to the desired number of units. Be careful not to push the plunger back. It will contaminate the insulin. Withdraw the syringe. You're ready to inject.

5.   If necessary, clean injection site. You may have been told to clean the injection site with an alcohol swab. If the injection site is clean,

there's no need. A British study followed two groups of 5,000 people who gave themselves injections. One group used alcohol swabs, one didn't. There were only five infections and all of them were in the group that used alcohol swabs. Dr. Tim's sister, Kathy, who is a registered nurse was surprised to learn that some bacteria could grow in alcohol.

6. Inject. You're ready to inject the insulin. Gently pinch up a fold of skin. The fatty tissue just under the skin has fewer nerve endings than the muscle underneath it, so for some areas with less fat, you might want to inject at an angle. Once the needle is in, press the plunger down smoothly and steadily. Don't rush. Release the fold of skin and withdraw the needle. Break off or remove the needle and discard the syringe and needle properly. Never share your needles with anyone.

adjusting your insulin dosage

Understanding the way insulin works is the key to making wise use of your blood test information. If your blood glucose stays within the target range with your current dose, you probably don't need to change your dose very often, but there are good reasons to know how to adjust your insulin dose. You may be traveling and want flexibility in the timing of your meals and the foods you choose, or you'll want to know how to change your insulin dose if your blood glucose is too high or too low. You can't always get hold of your doctor or educator as quickly as you might like.

When you first start taking insulin, your doctor may change the dose several times based on your blood test results. Your initial insulin dose will be based on several factors, including your recommended carbohydrate intake. Carbohydrates affect the rise of blood sugar more than protein or fats. Don't be afraid to ask questions. Your doctor doesn't live with you every minute of the day, so you need to understand how your schedule of insulin works and why. As time goes by, you'll know how to adjust your insulin as knowledgeably as your doctor will.

When making changes, it's best not to adjust your insulin too frequently or too drastically. If possible, adjust your insulin one unit at a time. You can also use the 10 percent rule, adjusting a dose by approximately 10 percent of the total. If you take eight units of rapid- or short-acting at lunch, you'd adjust by one unit, since .8 units would be difficult to measure. If your overall blood tests are showing higher numbers, you can begin your adjustment by correcting your before-breakfast blood glucose. Your doctor or educator will help you understand how to do this. Once that's in the target range, then work to correct the lunchtime reading.

How will you know your insulin is working effectively? Altogether, class . . . BY TESTING! What's your goal? To bring your blood sugars as close to the target range of 80 to 120 before meals. You can be slightly higher, 120 to 140, before bed and two hours after eating.

These are goals you'll work toward, one blood test at a time. If you tend toward the Type A personality/perfectionist/control freak side of the map (territory I know well), please try not to have unrealistic expectations. With diabetes, every day is different. You're trying to reproduce an incredibly complex system that was designed by a superior intelligence. There are so many factors that affect your blood sugar: emotions, food, medication, hormones, exercise, temperature, and even altitude. A few higher than normal blood sugars are not a disaster. Your HbA1c, that measures your blood sugar over a ninety-day period, will give you the big picture.

long-acting holds the key

Getting the long-acting dose just right is an important key to good control. My friend Larry has had diabetes for thirty-seven years and has always been conscientious about controlling his blood sugar. He eats basically the same thing for breakfast and lunch everyday. He considers this approach his tradeoff for blood sugars that are consistently in the target range. By eating the same components for those two meals, he always knows exactly how much short-acting insulin to take at breakfast and lunch. A few years ago, his before-breakfast numbers started to rise. His doctor attributed it to the influence of the Dawn Phenomenon, a naturally occurring rise in early morning blood sugar.

Larry's educator recommended that he read *Stop the Rollercoaster* by John Walsh, Ruth Roberts, and Dr. Lois Jovanovic-Peterson. The book advised him to determine if his long-acting insulin was contributing to his blood sugar ups and downs. Larry tried an experiment and, for one day, took only long-acting insulin in the morning and then skipped breakfast and lunch. He didn't take additional short-acting insulin for those two meals. The idea was to see if the long-acting insulin was providing a basal rate to cover his basic metabolic needs before he even ate his meals. Based on his blood sugar readings that day, he adjusted the long-acting insulin dose so that his fasting blood sugar wasn't too high or too low during breakfast time and lunchtime. To quote the authors in *Stop the Rollercoaster*, "Setting up the long-acting insulin is the most important step in controlling the blood sugar."

After establishing his baseline need for long-acting, he looked at his short-acting insulin needs. Larry was surprised by this approach. He told me, "I don't know why they (his doctors) didn't figure this out before. Maybe they did, but nobody told me." In adjusting insulin, the emphasis is most often on the short-acting insulin taken before meals. Yet the action of longer-acting NPH does have some peaks (times of increased effectiveness) that can contribute to low blood sugar episodes.

This experiment inspired Larry to switch to Lantus that provides a slow, steady action for twenty-four hours without any peaks. He also began counting carbohydrates at his meals, which he hadn't done before. He'd always just "eyeballed" his meals and approximated his dose of short-acting insulin. In addition, for a few days, he tested his blood sugar both before and after his meals to check the accuracy of his carbohydrate counting with the action of the short-acting insulin. He was able to bring almost all his blood sugar tests in the target range.

When Dr. Tim starts a patient on insulin, he begins with 10 units of long-acting Lantus given before bed. The dosage of Lantus is then adjusted until the before-breakfast (fasting) blood sugar is in target range (80 to 120). He usually adjusts Lantus by 1 or 2 units at a time as each unit typically causes a drop in blood sugar of 30 to 50 points. Then he adds rapid-acting Humalog or Novolog before meals.

Work with your doctor and diabetes educator to determine the dosage of long-acting insulin to provide the perfect basal rate for your metabolism.

the 1800/1500 rules

If you are adjusting your before-meals insulin (Novalog, Humalog or Regular), you can use the 1800/1500 Rules to determine how many blood glucose points one unit of short-acting insulin will cover.

Dr. Paul Davidson developed the 1500 Rule to show how far your blood sugar will drop for every unit of Regular insulin you take. Because blood sugar tends to drop faster and farther on Humalog and Novolog insulins, the 1800 Rule is used for these insulins. (Some doctors use a 2000 Rule for these insulins.) These rules apply for anyone taking injected insulin.

Example: Let's say your blood sugar before lunch is 220. First, add up the total number of units of short-acting insulin you take during each day.

Let's suppose you take 10 units before each meal. That's 30 units for three meals. If you're using Regular insulin (the 1500 Rule), you divide 1500 by the total units, 30.

1500 divided by 30 = 50

That "50" means that each additional unit of Regular you take will lower your blood sugar by 50 points. With a before-lunch blood sugar of 220, two extra units of Regular insulin would lower your blood sugar 2 x 50 = 100 points, from 220 to 120, within your target range.

Example: If your blood sugar is 220 and your total Humalog (or Novolog) each day is 30 units, use the 1800 Rule:

1800 divided by 30 = 60.

Taking two extra units of Humalog or Novolog would lower your blood sugar by 2 x 60 =120 points, from 220 to 100, also within target range.

Once again, if you're using Regular, you use the 1500 Rule. If you use rapid-acting Humalog or Novolog, you use the 1800 Rule. Once you figure how much each unit lowers your blood sugar, that information will be accurate until you change your total daily dose of rapid- or short-acting insulin. Then you'll need to recalculate.

The 1800/1500 Rule allows you to set up an accurate personal sliding scale to lower unwanted high blood sugars. Discuss using it with your doctor or diabetes educator.

This table shows how these rules work.

Total Daily Insulin Dose	1800 Rule Point Drop per Unit of H or Novolog	1500 Rule Point Drop per Unit of Regular
20	90 mg/dl	75 mg/dl
25	72 mg/dl	60 mg/dl
30	60 mg/dl	50 mg/dl
35	51 mg/dl	43 mg/dl
40	45 mg/dl	38 mg/dl
50	36 mg/dl	30 mg/dl
60	30 mg/dl	25 mg/dl
75	24 mg/dl	20 mg/dl
100	18 mg/dl	15 mg/dl

Adapted from *Insulin Pump Therapy Handbook*, copyright © 1992 John Walsh, P.A., C.D.E. and Ruth Roberts, M.A.

waiting

Letting some time elapse between your shot and eating your meal is another way to fine-tune blood sugar control. Waiting gives short-acting Regular time to start working before more food/glucose is poured into the bloodstream. You can use waiting instead of taking additional insulin to bring your blood sugar down. You need to tailor your waiting time to the insulin you're using and the level of your blood sugar reading. For example, Regular begins working in 20 to 30 minutes, so if your blood sugar is 120 to 150, you might wait 30 minutes; 150 to 200, you'd wait 45 minutes. If it is over 200, you might wait 60 minutes. Discuss recommended waiting times for the insulin you're taking with your doctor or educator.

If you are using Humalog or Novolog, don't wait to eat. A fifty-year-old patient of Dr. Tim's took his Humalog and was ready to eat dinner when the doorbell rang. Some friends had stopped by for a visit. Instead of eating he talked with them until thirty minutes later, when he began speaking gibberish. His wife gave him fruit juice and a cookie, and then checked his blood sugar. It was still too low. She injected glucagon into his stomach and it brought his blood sugar into the normal range so that he was able to function again. He had wanted to be polite to his company, but that night he decided if that circumstance happened again, he would excuse himself and eat his dinner first.

If your blood sugar is high before a meal, why wait? Why not just take more insulin? Insulin is adipogenic: it helps the body store fat. That's one of the reasons it can be so difficult for those who inject insulin to lose weight. The ideal is for you to take as little insulin as necessary to achieve good blood sugar control. Having said that, I would add that it is essential to take as much insulin as is needed to achieve good blood sugar control. Don't ever sacrifice good control by using less insulin than you need.

insulin reactions

We'll cover the fine points of blood sugar control in Chapter Nine, but here are the basics about insulin reactions. They occur when you have more insulin in your system than you need. Insulin takes sugar out of your bloodstream, either sending it into your cells or tucking it away as fat, so the more insulin you take, the lower your blood sugar. When your blood sugar falls below the normal range, your brain will not be getting enough fuel. You might feel dizzy, hungry, confused, or shaky, among other symptoms. If the blood sugar drops really low, you could lose consciousness or have a convulsion, so it's important to treat low blood sugar quickly.

If this happens to you and you still have your wits about you, do a blood test so you know exactly where you are. Treat a low blood sugar with glucose tablets, or a small glass of juice or sugared soda, followed by a small serving of protein, fat and carbohydrate, such as cheese and crackers or half a sandwich, to help stabilize your blood sugar. After 15 minutes, you can test again to see if you're in the normal range.

Plan for your exercise sessions. Exercise burns glucose, making insulin more effective. In order to avoid an insulin reaction during exercise, you need to look at the time your insulin will be reaching its peak efficiency and the timing of your exercise sessions. For example, a tennis game at 3:00 in the afternoon will occur just as NPH is peaking. If you know you'll be playing that afternoon, you'd want to consider taking a little less NPH that morning or eating an extra snack before you play, or both. Also long periods of strenuous exercise can result in lower insulin needs for eight to sixteen hours. That means you could get a reaction in the afternoon from a morning soccer game. Your doctor and diabetes educator can help you plan for these occasions.

dawn phenomenon and somogyi effect

If you find yourself waking up with high blood sugar, it could be due to special circumstances. The Dawn Phenomenon is caused by a natural release of growth hormone and cortisol during the early morning hours. Growth hormone and cortisol cause the liver to release glucose, resulting in a high morning blood sugar. It's theorized that this rise is a holdover from the days when humans would go out for the hunt early in the day. Or perhaps it's just the body's way of helping us get the day started! Whatever the cause, for some people this phenomenon creates an additional difficulty with blood sugar control.

If you're using conventional therapy with only two shots a day, giving a third shot of NPH right at bedtime, say at 10:00 P.M., can help lower this early morning rise, as NPH or Lente peaks approximately seven to eight hours later. This may allow you to "sleep in" an extra hour or two and still have control of your fasting blood glucose.

Lantus taken at night can also help neutralize the Dawn Phenomenon. To determine if you are on the proper dose of Lantus, you should have control of your fasting (before breakfast) blood sugar. If your fasting blood sugar is high, over 120, then you may need extra Lantus at bedtime.

The Somogyi Effect is the name given to the rebound from an untreated low blood sugar to a high blood sugar. It's most likely to happen at night. Because you're asleep, you're not likely to notice the symptoms of low blood sugar: dizziness, confusion, and shakiness. If your low blood sugar goes untreated for a period of time, the liver releases glucagon to force the body to release stored energy. The glucagon raises your blood sugar, sometimes above the target range.

You can determine if your blood sugar is rebounding by waking at 3:00 A.M. and taking your blood sugar. If it's normal or a little on the low side at 3:00 A.M. and then high in the morning, you're probably rebounding. It means you're taking more insulin at night than you need, which is lowering your blood sugar too much. This is most likely to occur if you take NPH rather than Lantus.

If you're having high before-breakfast readings, ask your doctor and educator to help you adjust your nighttime insulin dose. If it's the Dawn Phenomenon, you may need a little more long-acting insulin. If it's the Somogyi Effect, you may need either less short- or long-acting in the evening shot.

Does all this information feel a bit overwhelming? One of Dr. Tim's patients told him, "Yesterday I was diagnosed with diabetes. Today I need to know ten thousand new things!" He had looked through several books on diabetes and felt that he had to learn everything all at once. By his third diabetes education class, he was starting to get the hang of things and commented, "Diabetes is an aggravation, but it's easier than my job." (He was an electrical engineer who usually worked sixty to eighty hours a week.)

I remember feeling as if I'd never learn all I needed to know to properly care for my son. I did, Brennan did, and so will you. During these early weeks of learning about diabetes, it's vital that you have consistent access to your doctor and/or your diabetes educator. Also, a diabetes mentor who takes insulin can help your understanding by sharing his or her own experiences. Your local diabetes organization may help you connect with someone through a support group. With time, experience, and patience, you will be surprised how much you'll learn about caring for your own diabetes and how quickly.

The idea that helped most . . . was to remember that the foods I wasn't eating were not leaving the planet.

chapter six

food, glorious food

A few years ago, my mother passed on. I watched her decline for seven years, yet at the same time, my health was improving, largely because of her. Fifteen years before, she had visited me. One evening, as she stood at the sink washing the dinner dishes, I noticed how stooped her posture was. I realized that just as I had absorbed some of her other traits and tendencies, I was probably going to have the same stooped posture if I didn't do something about it. I began going to yoga classes. My posture, as well as my strength and flexibility, improved.

I began making healthier choices, but I couldn't get my mother to accept the idea that the choices she made each day affected her health. I watched her spend the last 10-percent of her life in a wheelchair. Her disabilities were almost all caused by lifestyle choices.

At the health club where I teach yoga, I overheard someone say, "You are what you do everyday." I know it's true. I see students who take yoga even twice a week improve their strength, balance, and flexibility. We are born with and develop certain tendencies, yes, but that doesn't mean we have to be a victim of those tendencies. The body is remarkably resilient, but we have to give it the raw materials to accomplish good health, every day, every week. It's the drip, drip, drip of water that wears away stone and it's the drip, drip, drip of high-calorie, high-fat foods, stressful thoughts, and lack of movement that wears down the body's ability to repair itself and ward off disease.

I know I don't want to follow in my mother's health footsteps. So what do I want? I want to be the healthiest person I know the day before I die. I realize that the choices I make every day either increase or decrease my health resources. I ask myself, "Did I do one hour of exercise today?" I don't do it every day, but I remind myself of that goal. When I go to the refrigerator, I often ask, "What do I want?" I don't mean what food do I want, I mean what outcome do I want? Standing there with the fridge door open, I have a moment of choice. I want health, so I most often choose food that provides high quality nourishment. I don't always make perfect choices, but asking the question, "What do I want?" and answering, "I want good health," helps reinforce my commitment to myself.

The suggestions in this chapter present the biggest challenge of living with diabetes. They ask you to transform your relationship with food. Controlling blood sugar is a constant challenge of balancing medication, movement, and food. Many adults who get diabetes take their medication and may even do some exercise, but most admit that changing their eating patterns is a big struggle. You may not have thought too much about your eating patterns before now. Diabetes demands you pay attention to when you eat, what you eat, and how much you eat.

Scott has learned to do that since he was diagnosed. He lives in the country and his family grows much of their own food, but Scott never liked to eat the way the rest of his family did. While they were eating lots of fruits and vegetables fresh from the garden, Scott would fix himself a frozen pasta dish or barbecue a steak or hamburger. He even had a section of the cupboard reserved for his cookies and candy. His body reflected his choices. He was eighty pounds overweight and tested positive for diabetes. His triglycerides were high, his HDL (good) cholesterol was low, and he had high blood pressure. These are all markers for what health professionals call "metabolic syndrome." Metabolic syndrome leads to diabetes, heart attacks, strokes, and vascular disease. With education and support, he's gradually learning to change his eating patterns. He's sharing his family's healthy meals, losing weight, and getting his diabetes under control.

This chapter is going to give you the information you need to make good choices. I hope you'll be well informed on this subject by your doctor and diabetes educator. Perhaps you'll even have access to a dietitian. If so, this information will supplement materials they give you. The good news is that you'll not be asked to follow some strange diet that will isolate you from the rest of the world. The diabetes food plan you'll be asked to adopt contains the same healthy recommendations outlined by the American Heart Association and the American Cancer Society.

As a person with diabetes, you'll be asked to consume the amounts of food that keep your blood sugar in the target range and to plan your meal times to match the action of your diabetes medications. If you're overweight, you may be counseled to lose weight. Losing weight will decrease your insulin resistance, making it easier to control your blood sugar levels. It can also help lower your blood pressure and reduce your risk of heart disease and may reduce or eliminate the need for diabetes medications.

your dining experience

There's so much conflicting information about food these days. No one likes to hear the "d" word . . . diet. Yet every one of us is on a diet. In the dictionary, "diet" is defined as "what a person usually eats and drinks; daily fare."

So what's your daily fare? Radiant good health partially depends on eating nutritious meals. It's important that you give your body the nutrients it needs to maintain its functions.

Among these nutrients are:

◆ *Carbohydrates*—the source of energy found in bread, cereal, pasta, rice, legumes, fruit, starchy vegetables, and milk.

◆ *Protein* builds muscle and tissue and provides energy. It's present in animal sources—meat, poultry, fish, milk, cheese, and eggs—and plant sources like tofu, legumes, grains, nuts, and some vegetables.

(continued on page 96)

- *Fat* is the storage form of energy and is found in oils, butter, margarine, mayonnaise, salad dressing and gravy, meat, dairy products, nuts, avocados, olives, seeds, peanut butter, baked goods, chips, crackers, and snack foods. Fats are often a hidden factor in prepared foods and restaurant foods.
- *Vitamins* are complex organic compounds that help your body function correctly.
- *Minerals* help control the body's water balance, hormones, and fluids.
- *Water*, which makes up a large portion of your body, is vital to good health. Active people require two quarts of water a day. If your blood sugar is elevated, or if you drink caffeinated beverages, you need extra water. Caffeine is a diuretic. If you have a heart problem, check with your doctor about how much water you should drink.

There are countless books on diet and health, but I think there are three essential instructions for a healthy perspective on food. These points apply to those of us who have diabetes and those who don't.

1. *Eat a variety of healthy foods.*

Focus on the positives and include foods that build health each day. Try to include two to three servings of fruit and three to four servings of vegetables a day. Eyeball a serving by imagining the amount that would fit in the palm of your hand. Not the whole hand with fingers, just the palm. That's one serving.

My friend, Deborah, who's had diabetes for forty years, says, "I try to eat from a positive viewpoint. I have fruit with every meal and always carry fruit such as an apple with me. That way I know I get good nutrition from the fruit and it also helps fill me up. At lunch and dinner I always have at least two servings of vegetables, including a salad."

Larry has had diabetes for thirty-seven years and also approaches food from an inclusive viewpoint. He always eats fruit with breakfast and lunch, and has lots of vegetables at dinner.

There are a few other simple directives that really help bring you toward healthier habits. Choose broiled, baked, and roasted protein sources. Take the skin off the chicken and turkey and cut the fat off red meat. Eat fish once or twice a week. I'm sure you've also heard about staying away from fried foods, eating whole grains, and choosing lean meats and poultry. Those are all great ideas.

Deborah advises, "Make it simple for yourself by getting into a daily routine and committing yourself to having healthy habits. Don't think about what you can't be doing; think about what you can be doing. Take pleasure in what you're eating. I look at every meal as a 'dining experience.' My co-workers tease me about this, saying 'What's going to be our dining experience today?'"

2. Be consistent.

Eat about the same amount of food at the same time each day. My doctor recently mentioned that this helps keep the rhythm of hunger and digestion.

Larry's focus is on consistency. "Regarding diabetes and what I eat, staying healthy is most important to me. I find that for breakfast and lunch I eat pretty much the same thing every day. Breakfast is always Shredded Wheat sweetened with Equal, a sliced banana, and low-fat milk. Lunch is a sandwich of turkey and cheese with lettuce on whole wheat bread, a piece of fruit, and a glass of juice. I've found that the juice and fruit help prevent an afternoon low blood sugar."

Larry allows himself more freedom at dinner. At the beginning of the week, he makes a pot of stew or chicken soup with lots of vegetables and it's there for him anytime he needs it. Any night he's not going out with friends, he has stew or soup and a piece of bread for dinner.

Larry says, "Being consistent with my food intake allows me to see what other things affect my blood sugar, such as exercise and emotional or mental activity. When I'm teaching, I use a lot of energy. It's mental energy, yet it affects my blood sugar as much as a workout at the gym. The days when I don't teach, I can see the difference in my blood sugar readings. When I'm teaching, I know I need to reduce my insulin or eat a little more. I like to keep my meals about the same, so I usually choose to adjust the insulin."

There are rewards for consistency. Deborah says, "My payback is that I feel better when I eat healthy, nutritious food."

Larry agrees, "The positive side of having this kind of discipline is that I get a healthy, pretty normal life. It's the same discipline I've had to have as a musician. In order to play my very best, I had to practice every day for many years and now I have the freedom to enjoy the results of my efforts. I look at diabetes in the same way, as a kind of blessing. If I didn't have diabetes to point me in the right direction, I might not have made the effort to have such a balanced life. I'm grateful for that."

One diabetes educator's client told her, "Diabetes has probably saved my life. I knew I needed to make some lifestyle changes and diabetes made me do that."

3. *Allow for flexibility.*

Diabetes is not about deprivation; it's about moderation. There's a time and a place for everything. A young woman called her diabetes educator in tears because she thought she couldn't attend a friend's wedding. She said, "I can't go. There will be cake. I know I'll be too tempted and it will spoil the whole day for me." Her educator convinced her she could have a small piece of cake by adjusting her insulin dosage.

Larry uses this approach. "I think you really have to find your own way with all of it. That includes testing your blood sugar, taking your medication, and experimenting with the way different foods affect you. For example, diary products don't greatly affect my blood sugar. I can eat cheese and drink milk and I'm fine, but pizza and pasta really elevate my readings. Of course, they're very high in carbohydrates. Also, Chinese food and Thai food are red flags for me. Thai food has a lot of hidden sugar in the sauces. I enjoy Mexican food, which is also high in carbs. If I'm going out with friends to an ethnic restaurant, I know I'll need to take more insulin. With observation and patience, each of us can discover what works."

Larry notes, "It's not that I never have a 'treat.' Sometimes there's a last minute choice like, 'Dad, let's go play racquetball.' Perhaps I've already taken my insulin at lunch, so I know I have to eat something extra. That's when I choose a cookie or some regular ice cream (not diet). It gives me the extra boost I need."

♦ ♦ ♦

the big three and their entourage

All the foods you eat can be assigned to one of three nutrient categories: carbohydrates, protein, and fat. Fat has 9 calories per gram, and protein and carbohydrates each have 4 calories per gram. Fat has more than twice the calories of protein and carbohydrates. Let's look at carbohydrates first.

carbohydrates

Carbohydrates are the body's primary source of energy and are commonly known as sugars and starches. There are two kinds of carbohydrates: simple and complex. Simple carbohydrates are sugars that break down very quickly. There are several kinds; lactose, found in milk; glucose and fructose, found in fruits and vegetables; and sucrose, what we know as table sugar. These sugars are found in a wide variety of foods—fruit, fruit juice, fruit drinks, milk, ice cream, frozen yogurt, sherbet, syrup, honey, molasses, jam and jelly, pies, cakes, cookies, donuts, sweetened soft drinks, and candy.

Complex carbohydrates are made up of a large number of sugar molecules that join together in a long chain. They're found in the starches we eat—bread, pasta, rice, beans, potatoes, etc. Foods with fiber, like whole grains, fruits, and vegetables, are also complex carbohydrates.

The body breaks down all carbohydrates into glucose. Then, in the presence of sufficient insulin, the glucose enters the cells to be used for energy or it's stored for future use. For years it was accepted that simple carbohydrates entered the bloodstream faster than complex carbohydrates, but we now know that's not the case. It's generally accepted that all carbohydrates, whether simple or complex, are absorbed at about the same rate. That's why it's important for people with diabetes to pay attention to how much carbohydrate they eat. Yet carbohydrates do differ in how they affect the rise in blood sugar. We'll discuss that under the "Glycemic Index" section.

It's recommended that most of your carbohydrate choices come from the complex carbohydrate group. Complex carbohydrates are excellent sources of nutrition and fiber. Fiber helps slow down digestion, so the blood sugar rises more slowly and consistently. Complex carbohydrates include whole grains and cereal products, most vegetables, and legumes.

fiber in carbohydrates

Fiber is plant material that cannot be digested by humans. It's found in unrefined grains (whole wheat, brown rice, corn, millet, barley, etc.) and dried beans, peas, fruits, and vegetables. Fiber content is an important factor in choosing carbohydrate foods. Foods high in fiber fill you up, taking up space in your stomach and intestines, absorbing water, and slowing down digestion so that you feel full longer. In the large intestine, fiber helps eliminate solid waste and is recommended to reduce the risk of colon cancer. High fiber foods also help lower blood pressure and decrease blood fat levels. Fiber-rich foods such as oats, beans, and whole-grain breads seem to increase the body's sensitivity to insulin and can sometimes lower a person's insulin requirements.

There are many ways to increase the fiber in your diet:

✦ Eat a lot of vegetables (at least two cups/day). Choose fresh vegetables with edible skins and seeds. Scrub, don't peel, the carrots. Leave the skins on the potatoes. Steam vegetables with the skins on.

✦ Choose whole fresh fruit instead of fruit juice.

✦ Choose whole-grain products in their natural coatings. Choose brown rice instead of white, converted rice instead of instant. Use whole-wheat bread, spaghetti and noodles, whole-wheat tortillas and crackers, and whole-grain cereals like oatmeal.

✦ Use cooked dried beans, peas, and lentils as a carbohydrate source. They have no cholesterol, contain both protein and carbohydrate, and are an excellent fiber source to help lower cholesterol.

✦ Read the cereal labels. As a general rule, the shorter the list of ingredients, the more nutritious the product. Look for whole grain listed as the first ingredient, with no added sugar.

✦ Eat flaxseed. Grind 1 tbsp. before each meal in a coffee grinder and eat with cereal or vegetables to help lower cholesterol and increase soluble fiber intake. Flaxseed also contains beneficial fats.

✦ Sprinkle a tablespoon of oat bran or wheat germ over salads, hot cereal, or cottage cheese.

✦ Add wheat germ, ground flaxseed, or oat bran to meatloaf and meatballs.

If these suggestions are new to you, increase your fiber intake gradually to avoid bloating and gaseous discomfort. Also, drink eight to twelve glasses of non-caffeinated fluid, preferably water, each day to prevent added fiber from causing constipation. If you have a history of heart disease, you should check with your doctor about the amount fluid you should have.

low carb vs. high carb

There's an ongoing controversy about whether people with diabetes should be eating a low carbohydrate or high carbohydrate diet. *The Diabetes Food and Nutrition Bible*, published by the American Diabetes Association, tells us to "make starches the star." It suggests that a high carbohydrate diet of 60 percent grains, beans, and starchy vegetables should be the foundation of an eating plan of a person with diabetes.

Then there's Dr. James Anderson of Veteran's Administration Hospital in Lexington, Kentucky. He takes the ADA's diet one step further by adding a special emphasis on fiber. His approach has had consistent success in lowering insulin requirements, blood pressure and cholesterol levels, and improving blood glucose control. Insulin doses for Type 1 patients in one of his research studies decreased by 38 percent and for Type 2 by 58 percent. His program also resulted in 52 percent of obese Type 2 participants being taken off insulin completely.

The carbohydrate foods included in the HCF plan are all high in fiber and nutrition. They're whole grains, beans, starchy vegetables like squash and corn, non-starchy green and orange vegetables, fruits, nonfat milk, extra-lean protein, and healthy fats. The fiber content is supplied by eating foods with their natural fibrous coating: brown rice instead of white; whole grains like oats, bran, and cracked wheat; whole fruits instead of juices. The diet gives you 30 to 60 grams of fiber a day. Dr. Anderson has found that compliance for this diet has been good. The high fiber content promotes the feeling of fullness after eating, and the low glycemic index foods in this diet supply a slower rise in blood sugar that contributes to improved blood sugar control for many people.

Most of the foods you eat with his plan are the ones richest in vitamins, minerals, and antioxidants. These nutrients are highly recommended by all health experts to protect against cancer and heart disease. It seems that eating foods high in fiber also helps prevent diabetes. Not too many years ago, the inhabitants of a tiny island changed their diet from their locally grown, high-fiber foods to low-fiber meats and processed foods imported from abroad. Thirty percent of the inhabitants over the age of fifteen now have diabetes. For more information about the HCF plan, go to www.hcf-nutrition.org.

There are experts who disagree with a high carbohydrate diet. Dr. Richard Bernstein, author of *Diabetes Solution*, has had Type 1 diabetes for fifty-seven years and he is adamant that a low carb diet is most beneficial. In the 1970s, failing health caused him to wonder why people with diabetes were advised to eat a diet that is basically 50 to 60 percent sugar. In a recent article in *U.S. News and World Report*, Dr. Lois Jovanovic-Peterson, chief scientific officer of Sansum Medical Research Institute called diabetes a disease of "carbohydrate intolerance" and stated that diabetes meal plans should minimize carbohydrates. Some people find that lowering their intake of carbohydrates can significantly improve their blood sugar control. As we mentioned in Chapter Five, the amount of insulin you take is largely determined by how your body reacts to the carbohydrates you eat. The confusion here is that while it's true that the body converts both simple and complex carbohydrates into simple sugars, carbohydrate foods rich in natural fiber slow the rise in blood sugar after a meal and provide a wealth of essential nutrition.

There are strong opinions on both sides of this debate, but what matters most is how your body responds to the carbohydrates you eat. Your blood tests will tell you the story. Say you go out for dinner and find that two pieces of pizza result in a high blood sugar a few hours later. Pizza is mostly made of processed white flour and tomato sauce, higher glycemic index foods. You could contrast that blood sugar result with what happens after a meal containing the same number of carbohydrates from lean meat, fresh vegetables, and whole grains or beans. Aside from the fact that the second dinner provides better overall nutrition, it most likely will result in much better blood test numbers.

If you're following the current standard of 50 to 60 percent of your calories from carbs and are having trouble controlling your blood sugar, take a look at the kind of carbs you're eating. Are they high in natural fiber and low on the glycemic index? Talk with your health professional about shifting the emphasis of your eating plan to include more whole grains, beans, vegetables, and fruits. You can also discuss moving toward a lower carb diet by replacing some of the starchy carbs with a little more protein and healthy fats from monounsaturated oils, avocado, and nuts.

Learning to count the amount of carbohydrate in each meal will be very helpful to good blood sugar control. Your educator will work with you to set your recommended daily carbs. Then you can get a guide such as the ADA's *Complete Guide to Carb Counting* by Hope Warshaw, M.M.S.c, R.D., C.D.E., B.C.-A.D.M. and Karmeen Kulkarni, M.S., R.D., C.D.E., B.C._A.D.M. or *Dr. Atkins' NEW Carbohydrate Gram Counter*. Knowing how to count carbs will give you the flexibility to manage your blood sugar while enjoying a wide variety of foods.

protein

Protein builds and repairs the body's tissue and can also be used as energy. The word protein comes from a Greek word meaning "of first importance." Protein is comprised of a chain of amino acids. There are twenty-two amino acids you need for survival, but the body only manufactures thirteen of them. The other nine must come from the foods you eat.

We need moderate amounts of protein from animal or vegetable sources each day. Protein is found in animal sources such as meat, poultry, fish, eggs, and milk products. Grains, legumes, and nuts also contain protein, as do some vegetables. One protein serving is approximately 3 ounces, the size of a deck of cards. Two to three protein servings (6-9 ounces) a day are enough for most people. Too much protein can cause elevated blood sugar and high cholesterol levels.

When you eat animal protein like chicken, fish, meat, or dairy products, the protein content is only part of the story. You might think that you're just having a serving of protein, but you may be getting a big serving of fat.

For example, an ounce of extra-lean meat has up to 1 gram of fat at 9 calories. That's only 9 calories of fat.

An ounce of lean meat contains up to 3 grams of fat at 9 calories per gram. That serving contains 27 calories of fat, three times as much as the extra-lean.

An ounce of medium fat meat has up to 5 grams fat at 9 calories for 45 calories of fat. That's five times the fat in the extra-lean serving.

An ounce of high-fat meat has up to 8 grams fat, times 9 equals 72 calories. That's eight times the fat of an extra-lean serving.

Here is how the protein choices compare:

♦ *Extra-lean:* approximately 35 calories and 1 gram fat per ounce
   Most fish (skinless), 1/4c. tuna in water, white-meat poultry, 1/4c. low-fat cottage cheese, nonfat or 1 gram fat cheese, nonfat or 1 gram fat luncheon meats or hot dogs, 1/2c. legumes and dried beans

♦ *Lean:* 55 calories and 3 grams fat per ounce
   Salmon, 1/4c. tuna in oil, dark meat poultry, white meat poultry with skin, 1/4 c. cottage cheese, 1/4c. cheese with 3 grams fat, lean beef like sirloin or flank steak, processed ham, veal chop or roast, 2T. Parmesan cheese

♦ *Medium-fat:* 75 calories and 5 grams fat per ounce
   Most pork, most beef, trimmed prime rib, lamb, corned beef, poultry with skin, fried fish, fried poultry, cheeses with 5 grams fat, mozzarella and ricotta cheese, eggs

♦ *High-fat:* 100 calories and 8 grams of fat per ounce
   Prime cuts of meat—untrimmed, spare ribs, regular cheese, sausages, hot dogs, bacon, and peanut butter

Each of these protein choices contains exactly the same amount of protein per ounce: 7 grams of protein at 4 calories for a total of 28 calories. Yet an extra-lean 3 oz. serving of meat gives you 105 calories, while a high-fat 3 oz. serving has 300 calories. That's 200 extra calories. If you have three servings a day and choose the extra-lean meat instead of high-fat each time, you've just eliminated 600 calories a day. Multiply that by 7 days and you've downsized your calorie intake each week by 4200 calories that could result in a one-pound weight loss each week.

fats and their co-horts

We hear so much about fat, low-fat and nonfat that many of us are confused. You may even think that fat is bad for you. Not true. Fat is necessary for good health. It helps maintain healthy hair and skin, and carries "fat-soluble" vitamins throughout the body. The body changes fats into fatty acids that are an energy source for the muscles and heart. Fat is also used to store energy.

Fat becomes a problem when we eat too much of it or eat the wrong kind of fat. In the average American diet, fat accounts for more than 40 percent of total calories. Fat and its partner, cholesterol, are culprits in two of our most deadly diseases, heart disease and cancer. Fat is a concern for those with diabetes because they have an increased risk of heart disease.

saturated fats

I'm sure you've heard of the importance of choosing beneficial fats. There are basically two kinds of fat: saturated and unsaturated. Saturated fat comes from animal sources such as meat, eggs, and dairy products and is generally solid at room temperature. The tropical oils, palm oil and coconut oil, are also saturated. (New studies suggest that they may not be as undesirable as animal sources of saturated fat.)

Saturated fats can narrow and block the blood vessels and contribute to heart disease, a major complication of diabetes. Saturated fats include butter, sour cream, cream cheese, coffee creamer, hard margarine, shortening, lard, palm and coconut oil, fried foods, bacon and sausage, gravy and cream sauce, and chocolate.

The fats found in fish are less saturated than animal fats and are, as a rule, good for you. Fish oil contains substances called Omega-3 long-chain fatty acids. Frequent consumption of these oils appears to be effective in reducing the risk of heart disease. Heart health experts recommend eating fatty fishes such as tuna, salmon, trout, and herring. Shellfish such as mussels, clams, scallops, and oysters are low-cholesterol foods as well. Caution: there are warnings out about eating certain fish because of high levels of mercury and other contaminants. Generally, it's been recommended that we buy fish from deep ocean waters or farm-raised fish, but even some of these are now undesirable for various reasons. Check with the butcher at your grocery store about which fish are currently safe.

Many of the processed foods we eat, like crackers, cookies, and some cereals, contain partially hydrogenated vegetable oil. It's a good idea to read labels of processed foods and try to avoid these oils. Hydrogenated oil has had its chemical structure changed and affects the body like a saturated fat. Some brands of peanut butter contain hydrogenated oil, so choose a brand that separates in the jar and doesn't have hydrogenated oil listed on the label. These hydrogenated oils contain "trans fatty" acids. More about that in a few pages . . .

unsaturated fat

Unsaturated fat comes from vegetables and is usually liquid at room temperature. They don't have an adverse affect on your blood vessels. Monounsaturates are found in olive and peanut oil and also in nuts, seeds, olives, and avocados. Monounsaturated fats are recommended because they are beneficial to the heart and cardiovascular system. They are the main fats used in Japan, Greece, and Italy where heart disease rates are very low. Polyunsaturated fats are found in safflower, sunflower, and corn oil, and should be used sparingly, as overuse of them has been associated with an increased risk of cancer.

All fats are high in calories and should be eaten in small amounts. Health officials have been emphasizing the need to decrease the total amount of fat in our diets. The percentage of dietary fat seems to be an important factor in the development of disease. A study of Japanese women found that when they lived in Japan and had a diet of less than 20 percent fat, they had a very low incidence of breast cancer. After moving to America and increasing their dietary fat intake to 25 to 30 percent, the incidence of breast cancer among these women was raised to our national level of one in ten.

Fat content in foods can be confusing. Until recently I didn't understand the enormous disparity between percentage of fat and percentage of fat calories. Do you know that 1 percent milk has 50 percent fewer fat calories than 2 percent milk? We'll discuss label reading later in this chapter, but here's a quick guide: every time you buy a packaged product, look at the grams of fat per serving. Multiply that number by 9. If the result is more than 25 percent of the total calories per serving, try to avoid that product.

To summarize the issue of fat: it's best to cut down your overall fat intake to under 30 percent. Some simple suggestions for doing this include: avoid butter most of the time, use margarine and oils sparingly, and avoid hydrogenated oils and lard whenever possible. When you use oil, choose monounsaturated ones like olive oil.

Other suggestions for cutting down on fat are:

+ Choose low-fat sources of protein, avoiding high-fat, high-cholesterol foods such as red meat, whole milk, butter, and whole-milk cheeses. When you do eat meat, choose lean cuts like sirloin or flank steak.
+ Stock your refrigerator with healthy choices like fresh fruits and vegetables.
+ Eat poultry and fish more often.
+ Trim off all visible fat before you cook. Remove the skin from poultry before you cook or cook with it on, but don't eat it.
+ Don't add fats in cooking. Broil, grill, boil, microwave, or bake rather than fry. If you do fry, use a little cooking spray and a non-stick frying pan.
+ Drink nonfat or 1 percent milk.

(continued on page 108)

- ✦ Eat no more than 2 to 4 eggs per week.
- ✦ Eat cheese sparingly or select cheese with less than 5 grams of fat per ounce.
- ✦ Use low-fat yogurt instead of cream, sour cream, and cream sauce.
- ✦ Mix nonfat sour cream with mayonnaise for sandwiches or salads.
- ✦ Flavor vegetables with herbs and spices instead of butter and sauces.
- ✦ Use lemon juice or vinegar on salads.
- ✦ Mix nonfat sour cream or plain yogurt with powdered ranch dressing mix to create a "free" dip or dressing.

cholesterol

Cholesterol is manufactured by the liver and the intestines, and acts in connection with fats in your body. Internally manufactured cholesterol is used in the formation of hormones, cell membranes, and protective sheaths for nerve fibers.

Cholesterol also enters the body in the foods we eat and takes a direct route to the blood vessels. Cholesterol buildup in blood vessels can lead to atherosclerosis, hardening of the arteries, which contributes to heart disease and strokes. Lowering dietary cholesterol is a good idea.

You help by eating foods low in cholesterol and by including a small amount of unsaturated fat each day. Exercise also helps increase your levels of "good" cholesterol. Most packaged products list the amount of cholesterol on the label. It's recommended that you eat no more than 300 milligrams per day.

trans fats

I've been interested in nutrition for a long time. Thirty years ago a healthy food magazine informed me that hydrogenated oils and "trans fatty acids" were bad for the body and heart. Back then those of us who were interested in good nutrition—whole grains, no trans fats, lots of vegetables—were called "health nuts." It's rather satisfying for me to read that experts now recommend the same "health nut" diet that was ridiculed not many years ago.

Most of us have heard that saturated fats are harmful to your body. Knowing this, we've switched from butter to margarine and have looked for labels that say "low-cholesterol" or "made with vegetable oil." Years of evidence proclaims that many of these so-called healthy foods have a substance hidden in them that does as much damage as saturated fats. The culprits are called trans fatty acids or trans fats.

Trans fats are formed when manufacturers take unsaturated fats that are in liquid form, such as corn oil, and put them through a process called hydrogenation. It makes the oil solid and more stable so it has a longer shelf life. This process of hydrogenation creates an artificial food with a molecule in it that the body doesn't recognize and is not easily metabolized. The body isn't able to break down and eliminate these fats and they damage the lining of our arteries. Dr. Tim repeats this admonition at the end of the book, but it bears saying here as well: if you see the words "partially hydrogenated" on the ingredient list, put that item back on the shelf. Why? Because studies show that trans fats increase the level of "bad" LDL cholesterol and suggest that trans fatty acids lower levels of "good" HDL cholesterol as well. In fact, studies indicate that trans fats may be implicated in almost 30,000 cardiac deaths a year. (That's a conservative estimate.)

I heard about the danger of trans fats thirty years ago, but it's taken all this time for that danger to be recognized and institutionalized by the experts. In the meantime, Americans have been eating trans fats. What's the lesson? Stay away from artificial food as much as you can. Food manufacturers are in business to make money, not to guard your health. It's your job to use common sense when it comes to the foods you eat. Your body was not designed to process artificial food and I have a feeling that many of the foods now touted as new diet solutions will be taken off the market as dangerous in the years to come.

Word has been getting out about the danger of trans fats, so many labels now claim, "No Trans Fats." If a packaged product doesn't mention those words, read the label.

alcohol

Alcohol is a drug that doesn't mix very well with diabetes. Some people with diabetes are able to drink alcoholic beverages in moderation, but you should carefully consider alcohol's relationship to your diabetes.

Alcohol contains no food values; it metabolizes as fat and has 7 calories per gram. Alcohol can contribute to nerve damage in the feet (neuropathy) with pain, tingling, and numbness, and it can make existing neuropathy worse. It can interfere with your diabetes medicines, and may cause pounding headaches, nausea, and a fast heartbeat. It often gives a false sense of confidence that makes it difficult to control the number of drinks taken. It can lower your blood sugar, causing extremely low blood sugar reactions in those using insulin or taking oral medications. That can be very dangerous, as people who see you drinking might think you're drunk when, in truth, you're having an insulin reaction and need immediate assistance.

If you're going to drink alcohol, moderation is the key. Limit yourself to one or two alcohol equivalents, preferably over a period of at least two hours. For most people, more than one drink per hour puts their blood alcohol level over the legal limit. An alcohol equivalent is a 4 oz. glass of wine, a 12 oz. light beer, or 1 1/2 oz. of hard liquor mixed with a sugarfree mixer.

Be certain to eat something if you're having a drink. Alcohol is absorbed directly from the stomach into the bloodstream, and then carried to the liver. While the liver is processing alcohol, it can't properly release stored sugar to assist with a low blood sugar. The blood sugar lowering effects of alcohol can last for up to thirty-six hours. Food in the stomach slows down the absorption of alcohol and reduces the amount of alcohol reaching the liver at any one time. Talk with your doctor and educator about alcohol use, and learn how to adjust your insulin or oral medication and your meal plan to make room for an occasional libation.

the glycemic index

Foods affect blood sugar differently. The graphs on p.111 illustrate how protein, carbohydrate, and fat impact blood sugar levels when eaten separately:

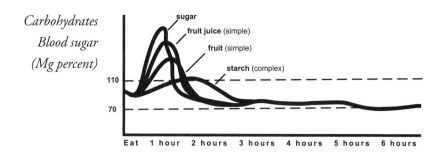

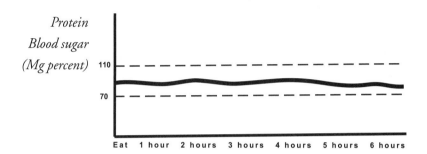

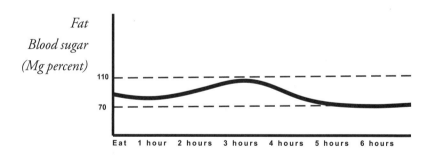

You can see that protein and fat (unless overeaten) keep the blood sugar fairly stable. Look again at the difference between the carbohydrates of sugar, fruit juice, fruit, and starches that contain complex carbohydrates. This variation is the reason that the glycemic index exists.

The glycemic index measures how much the blood sugar increases two to three hours after eating a carbohydrate food by itself. It compares the increase against a standard of 100 based on the increase caused by white bread or glucose, depending on the research study. There is a wide variation in biological response to foods such as fruit, corn, pasta, and bread. The lower the number on the glycemic index, the lower the rise in blood sugar.

Based on the 100 scale, here is how some foods rate:

Peanuts. 13	Sweet potatoes . . . 48	Brown rice 66
Lentils 29	Oatmeal 49	Shredded Wheat . . 67
Skim milk. 32	Pasta. 50	Mars Bars 68
Yogurt 36	Potato chips 51	White potatoes. . . 70
Ice cream 36	Green peas 51	White rice 72
Apples 39	Corn 59	Corn flakes. 80
Oranges 40	Bananas 62	Instant potatoes . . .80
Baked beans 40	Beets 64	Carrots. 92

Ice cream is low and carrots are high? That's a little confusing! That's the reason most doctors and educators don't even mention the glycemic index to their patients. Yet studies show that paying attention to the glycemic index may have value.

An article in the Journal of the *American Medical Association* reported the findings of the Nurse's Health Study of 121,700 female nurses. The study concluded that eating foods with a high glycemic index appeared to be a risk factor for Type 2 diabetes. Another study of 42,759 male health professionals showed that a high glycemic load also increased the risk of Type 2. High glycemic foods may prompt increased appetite. The journal *Pediatrics* reported that teenage boys ate nearly twice as much after a high glycemic index meal than after a low one.

The glycemic index is used in Canada, Australia, France, New Zealand, and the United Kingdom. Some dietitians in the U.S. have been reluctant to use it in a clinical setting, because each food is tested separately and we seldom eat a food all by itself. Yet we know that different carbohydrates give different responses. In her book, *Glucose Revolution*, Professor Jennie

Brand-Miller of Australia's University of Sydney details the differences in glycemia among six different mixed meals containing the same amount of carbohydrate, fat, and protein.

You can use the glycemic index to become more aware of foods that might send your blood sugar higher than normal. Ask your educator how you might effectively use the glycemic index ratings list.

sweeteners

There are two types of sweeteners: caloric and non-caloric. Table sugar, maple syrup, corn syrup, molasses, and honey are caloric sweeteners. Fructose is a naturally occurring sugar found in fruit and honey. People with diabetes should generally avoid these unless they are specifically planned into their diet.

Sorbitol, Mannitol, and Xylitol are naturally occurring alcohol sugars that cause a slower rise in blood sugar than table sugar, but which have the same number of calories. They are frequently used in diabetic ice cream, cookies, and candy. Their use is only recommended when blood sugar is in good control. When these products are consumed, minor intestinal problems, such as diarrhea, sometimes occur.

Saccharin is a non-caloric sweetener and is used in Sweet'NLow, Sugar Twin, and Weight Watchers sweeteners. They can be used for cooking and baking, but tend to have a bitter taste if too much is added. They're currently recognized as safe for use.

Aspartame, found in NutraSweet and Equal, is made from two amino acids that metabolize in the body as protein. It is 180 to 200 times sweeter than sucrose, so it takes very little for a sweet flavor. Aspartame is found in sugar-free products such as diet soda, dessert and topping mixes, powdered soft drinks, instant tea, cocoa mixes, and chewing gum. It's not recommended for baking, as it's unstable when exposed to heat. If aspartame is overheated, it turns into formalin and is thought to affect the nerves.

Cyclamates are available in Canada, but are banned in the United States because of suspected cancer-causing properties. Acesulfame-K, contained in Sunnette, is a low-calorie sugar substitute recently approved for use in cooking.

Splenda is a new sweetener that contains only a few calories. It's made of three sugars that are bonded together so the body can't separate them. It tastes like sugar and you can cook with it. Users report that about half as much is necessary compared with sugar even though the label says that 1 tsp. = 1 tsp. of sugar.

Stevia is an excellent non-caloric sweetener made from a plant that is up to 300 times sweeter than sugar. It's available in health food stores as powder, pills, and diluted liquid.

Because they don't raise blood sugar very much, sugar substitutes are acceptable to use with your diabetes meal plan, but they're no help if you're having a low blood sugar. That's when you get to enjoy that chocolate chip cookie you've been thinking about!

reading food labels

The government requires that all packaged foods carry a label with certain basic information about the food inside and its nutrient content. Many products are labeled "Light," "Low fat" and "Cholesterol Free." These claims can only be used if the food meets strict government definitions. They are:

✦ Calorie free means the food contains less than 5 calories.
✦ Low Calorie means 40 calories or less.
✦ Reduced calorie—contains 25 percent fewer calories per serving than the usual product.
✦ Diabetic or Sugar Free—may contain a substitute sugar acceptable for diabetics. Read the label. The grams of carbohydrate per serving should be less than 5 grams.
✦ Diet or dietetic food has been changed in some way. It is important to read the label. Dietetic may mean the product is low in sodium, fat, or cholesterol, but not always low in sugar.
✦ Lite, Light, Sugar-Free, or No Added Sugar—use caution with these labels. Light can mean one of three things: the product contains one-third fewer calories or half the fat of the regular

product, the sodium (salt) content has been reduced by one-half, or it can be a description of the color or texture of the product.

✦ The word "sugar" on labels means "white sugar" only. All other types of sugars and sweeteners will be listed separately.

✦ Light in Sodium means 50 percent less sodium.

✦ Fat free means less than 1/2 gram of fat.

✦ Low fat means 3 grams or less fat.

✦ Cholesterol free means less than 2 milligrams cholesterol and 2 grams or less saturated fat.

✦ Sodium Free means less than 5 milligrams sodium.

✦ Very Low Sodium means 35 milligrams or less sodium.

✦ High Fiber means 5 grams or more fiber.

As a person with diabetes, reading labels and knowing how to interpret what you're reading are important skills. Let's take a quick look at two containers of yogurt: Yoplait Original and Yoplait Light.

The Yoplait Original label says it's 99 percent fat free—sounds good, right? Yet the label lists sugar as the second ingredient, then modified cornstarch, then high fructose corn syrup. That's three sources of starch and sugar out of the top four ingredients. It contains 33 grams of carbohydrate and 170 calories. Remember our graphs about blood sugar rise? Carbs affect the rise of blood sugar much more than protein or fat.

In comparison, Yoplait Light has 20 grams of carbohydrate and 110 calories. It lists high fructose corn syrup, then modified cornstarch and aspartame (already defined above) as its sweeteners. With the smaller amount of caloric sugars and less carbohydrates, the Yoplait Light would be a better choice.

The words *fat free, natural,* and *light* can be misleading. I bought some microwave popcorn this week that advertised "Natural Flavor" on the box. I neglected to read the label, thinking that since it was a microwave product it would be low in fat. I took one package out last night and noticed that the two main ingredients are popcorn and partially hydrogenated vegetable oil, which means trans fatty acids. And half the calories of each serving are from fat. That product is now in my garbage can. Better there than in my body.

a pyramid a day . . .

I first became familiar with the concept of food exchanges after I had my second child, Robin. I needed to lose twenty pounds and tried Weight Watchers. When Brennan was diagnosed with diabetes two years later, the American Diabetes Association's Exchange Diet seemed like an old friend. It divides food into categories or classes depending on the protein, carbohydrate, and fat content. The idea is that each food has approximately the same composition and caloric content as others in its class. This concept of grouping foods is utilized for several different systems used by dietitians and educators.

Every five years, the U.S. Department of Agriculture (USDA) and the Department of Health and Human Services release dietary guidelines that provide nutritional advice to Americans. The USDA's current Food Guide Pyramid (issued in 2005) emphasizes six major food groups that are close to the generally accepted food exchanges. It highlights the importance of grains, fruits, and vegetables, over the meat and dairy food groups. The USDA's guidelines are the most widely used and also urge Americans to be physically active and maintain a healthy weight. Dr. Meir Stampfer, Professor of the Departments of Epidemiology and Nutrition, and Chair of the Department of Epidemiology at Harvard School of Public Health, served on the committee for the 2000 and 2005 guidelines. Dr. Stampfer is a world-renowned investigator whose research has shown strong associations between dietary and other lifestyle modifications and the prevention of disease. He believes the current recommendations have not incorporated the latest research.

For the past two decades, recommendations have emphasized consuming more carbohydrates in place of fats. Many studies have provided evidence that not all fats are bad and not all carbohydrates are good. Dr. Stampfer says that whole grain sources of carbohydrates are good, but that at the recommended 6 to 11 servings per day, the carbohydrate category is overemphasized.

He says the same of the dairy category. He believes that Americans should be eating more fruits and vegetables and fewer dairy products. We've heard that it's necessary to get adequate amounts of calcium to prevent osteoporosis, yet Dr. Stampfer and his colleagues have found that greater consumption of milk and dairy products does not substantially protect against hip and forearm fractures. It's also been found that high calcium intake may increase the risk of cancer. There are other differences between the USDA's Pyramid and The Harvard Healthy Eating Pyramid. Differences in the Harvard model include the following recommendations:

✦ Whole grains, vegetable oils, fruits, and vegetables are emphasized.

✦ Physical activity and weight control are emphasized.

✦ Red meat and refined grains (white bread and white rice) are de-emphasized and listed as ingredients to be eaten sparingly.

✦ Nuts and legumes receive their own category.

✦ Dairy products are de-emphasized and placed in a category with calcium supplements.

✦ A daily multivitamin tablet is recommended for most people and daily moderate alcohol intake is a healthy option unless it does not make sense for that individual.

The Harvard Healthy Eating Pyramid looks like this:

Illustration: adapted from Eat, Drink, and Be Healthy *by Walter C. Willett, M.D.*

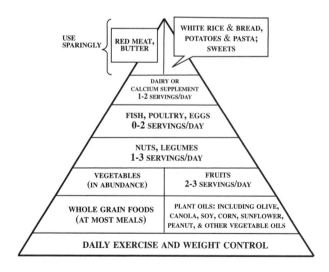

To see how your choices compare with these dietary recommendations, you might write down everything you eat for one week. Don't try to change anything, just take notes. You may be surprised by what you see. A woman who was certain she ate very little complained that no matter what she did, she could never lose weight. When she wrote down everything she put into her mouth, she was shocked to see how the calories added up. It was true that she hadn't been eating very much at meals, but she was snacking almost every hour as she was walking around the house. I used to kid my girlfriends that eating Häagen-Dazs doesn't count if it never hits the bowl. Oh, I wish it were true.

Once you see what you're actually eating, you can begin to think about what could be changed for the better. Perhaps you're not eating fresh fruit. You could add one or two pieces a day and make the effort to do that for a week until it becomes a new habit. Then add whole-grain products. Look at the fat content of your meals and decide what could be better. You might spend one week trying to eat the recommended servings of vegetables. Concentrate on one food group at a time so that the shifts accumulate over a period of time. Your diabetes educator or dietitian can help you make these changes in your eating patterns.

a sample menu

I think it helps to have examples, so if we were planning one day's model menu, it might look like this:

Breakfast: A small piece of fruit—an apple, pear, or 1/2 banana
One cup whole grain cereal—oatmeal, Nutri-Grain, Total—with skim or 1 percent milk and non-caloric sweetener
Coffee or tea

Lunch: A sandwich with whole-grain bread and an unprocessed protein source such as grilled chicken or turkey breast, with lettuce and tomato, using mustard and just a quick swipe of mayonnaise, if you like
Two or three vegetable servings—carrot and celery sticks,

steamed broccoli, a small salad with a little olive oil and balsamic vinegar

A non-caloric beverage

A piece of fruit or fresh berries for dessert

Afternoon snack: An apple and string cheese or some walnuts

Dinner: Grilled or roasted lean meat or chicken or fish (One serving/3 oz. is the size of a deck of playing cards) Two or three servings of vegetables—preferably steamed or roasted (one serving is the size of a tennis ball) or a bowl of vegetable soup

One cup of carbohydrates (two servings)—winter squash, brown rice, a medium potato, corn and peas, beans, or lentils

Fruit for dessert

This sample menu would give you approximately six servings of starch/complex carbohydrates, three servings of lean protein, four servings of fruit, two servings of low-fat dairy, four to six servings of vegetables, and four to five fat servings. Most doctors and dietitians would be thrilled if their clients with diabetes ate this way. The servings of fruit and vegetables are the key to positive eating strategies. They help fill you up and provide valuable nutrition. Deciding to include them at every meal will help you focus on the benefits of healthy eating.

Your diabetes educator will give you information about food exchanges. You can use them to become more aware of the amount of carbohydrates you're ingesting at each meal. It's the carbohydrates that mainly affect the rise of blood sugar. Carbohydrates come from three main categories: dairy products, fruits, and the starch and bread group which includes bread, cereal products, and starchy vegetables such as potatoes, corn, beans, and peas. A serving of any of these foods has approximately 15 grams of carbohydrate (a dairy serving has 12 grams of carbohydrate).

Carbohydrate counting helps you keep track of the carbohydrates you eat during the day. It's an excellent method for getting blood sugar under control and anyone whose blood sugar is not within normal ranges can benefit from using it. People who take short-acting insulin at mealtimes and those on insulin pumps use carbohydrate counting to determine how much insulin they need. You can decide with your diabetes educator how many grams of carbohydrates to have at each meal. Then check your blood sugar two hours after your meal and see if it's close to the target range of 140 to 160 (the lower number is preferred.) If your levels are in that range then you know the carbohydrates you're eating and the medication or insulin you're taking are well matched. Talk with your educator about carbohydrate counting as a tool for blood sugar control.

queen of meal planners

Now that you have diabetes, you may have been told that it's important that you lose weight. That's true. Losing as little as 10–20 pounds can really improve your blood sugar control. As you lose weight, your diabetes medications may be decreased. Using diet and exercise, some people with Type 2 diabetes are able to restore the body to normal functioning, meaning normal blood sugars. This is a desirable accomplishment, because no matter how good your attempts at blood sugar control may, they will never be as good as what your body, without diabetes, can do. Changing lifelong patterns of eating is a big challenge. I know from experience.

My mother was the queen of meal planners. Her favorite topic of conversation was "the best brunch in town." She could go on and on about the restaurant that ran out of bagels during brunch. (Can you imagine—a brunch with no bagels?) After having survived a major heart attack, my mother opened her eyes long enough to gaze at us lovingly and whisper, "I'm hungry." When it was time to be released from the hospital, she got them to postpone her departure until mid-afternoon because, "They're having a really good lunch today." As I was growing up, the words "I'm starving" regularly whistled past my ears. Thankfully, none of my family has had any experience with starvation, but for us, hunger was an urgent matter. The occasions in my life when I've had to lose weight have not been easy. I love to cook and I love to eat, so I sympathize with anyone who's on a "diet."

Yet for too many of us, it's time for a wake-up call. America is suffering a major health crisis. We're making lifestyle choices that are wounding us, taking precious months and years from our lives. The number of Americans who are severely obese, meaning at least 100 pounds overweight, has quadrupled since 1996. Obesity foretells serious health consequences, including substantially higher rates of diabetes, high blood pressure, heart disease, stroke, cancer, arthritis, and back problems. There was a time when most of us lived close to the land. People had gardens or bought fresh local produce. They spent many hours a week in physical exertion, either working the land or using their bodies to get from place to place. People rarely ate between meals. This way of life has changed drastically for most of us, but the body still requires fresh, wholesome foods and movement to remain healthy. It is thrown out of balance by too many fats or sweets, or too much food, period.

At the same time we're getting fatter and fatter, we Americans are obsessed with weight loss. Bestseller lists are crowded with titles outlining the latest breakthrough diet plan. The problem isn't just losing weight, it's keeping it off. We find ourselves craving "comfort foods." There's a reason some foods feel comforting. They actually affect the chemistry of the brain.

The brain is made up of billions of nerve cells that are separated by gaps called synapses. Chemical messengers called neurotransmitters bridge these gaps. Serotonin is the most important of the forty known neurotransmitters for the regulation of appetite and sleep. A deficiency of serotonin produces carbohydrate craving, because carbohydrates temporarily boost serotonin levels. The problem is the calming effect of carbohydrates lasts only an hour or two. Then the cravings surface again.

Dr. Cal Ezrin, author of *Your Fat Can Make You Thin*, says, "Many overweight people admit that they get a lot of comfort from carbohydrate foods like chocolate, candy, cake, ice cream, soda, and so on. All these foods have the capacity to generate a little extra serotonin, the brain chemical that is responsible for a number of functions. Most importantly, it's the governor of the adequate quality of restorative sleep. I think serotonin and sleep are very closely related. You can't get people to stay on a reduced carbohydrate diet if they're short of serotonin. They will be like addicts. They will go for serotonin in the form of carbohydrates without any restraint, because this gives them comfort." Using this understanding, Dr. Ezrin outlines weight loss plans in his books, *The Type 2 Diabetes Diet Book* and *Your Fat Can Make You Thin.*

The food choices you make each day are contributing to your future health and functioning. That's always been the case, but now that you have diabetes, there's more urgency surrounding those choices.

not leaving the planet

The most vital aspect of your weight loss program is your motivation. You may want to wear certain clothes, or take part in activities, or just generally feel better. Once you find a good reason, stay focused on that positive goal. As you begin moving toward your goal, make a list of the benefits that you're starting to see and feel. Perhaps you're sleeping more soundly, feeling that you have more energy, or getting compliments on your appearance. Keep that list close by for the days or times when you feel discouraged. Remind yourself of how far you've already come. Some people keep a picture of how they did look (the most unflattering one they can find), so they don't forget where they were.

Many of us eat to fill up a hunger that has nothing to do with food. Maybe we're punishing ourselves for guilt over the past or out of boredom or depression. I have met several women who had been sexually molested as children and as adults realized they had chosen obesity to ward off any sexual notice. When they released and healed their past, they lost weight easily. If emotional eating is part of your life, a counselor or support group can help you address the underlying issues.

Whenever you're restricting your food choices, there's always a chance of feeling deprived. About ten years ago, I went on a special diet to rid myself of allergies. (It worked.) When I looked at the list of what I needed to avoid (which included citrus, apples, tomatoes, potatoes, eggplant, seafood, red meat, white flour, and more), my first reaction was, "What can I eat?"

Sometimes when we have to limit our food choices, we only notice what isn't on our plate. To counteract this perspective, make a list of all the foods you can have during your weight loss period. I read this in a book about raising children. They suggested dealing with picky young vegetable eaters (or non-eaters) by making a list of what they would eat and focus on those rather than nag about what they won't eat.

It's been shown that limiting our choices is a great way to lose weight. One study demonstrated that the more foods made available at a meal (such as at a buffet table), the more people overate. From the standpoint of digestion, it's advisable to eat only one kind of animal protein at a meal. My husband uses a simple technique to keep himself at normal weight: At each meal, he limits himself to one plate of food. He almost never goes back for second helpings.

The idea that helped most during my own diet dramas was to remember that the foods I wasn't eating were not leaving the planet. You might try reminding yourself that you can eat a certain food at another time, when your weight loss is accomplished. This concept helped me after my second son was born. I had twenty pounds to lose and was not eating any food made with white flour or sugar. One day someone brought me a plate filled with homemade brownies. The crisp smell of chocolate wafted up in front of me. It was torture. I told myself, "Gloria, they're not leaving the planet. Just because you can't have a brownie today doesn't mean you can't ever have one. You can have it when you're finished losing weight."

The math of losing weight is really simple. You need to burn more calories than you take in. You do that by eating less and moving more. The "moving more" part is really important, as reducing your calorie intake can slow your metabolism and regular exercise helps minimize metabolic slowdown.

I recently heard Dr. Phil McGraw talk with an obese woman who said she just couldn't seem to lose weight. As he questioned her, she mentioned that she ate three bags of corn chips each day. He remarked, "If you put down those chips, you'll lose 31 pounds this year!" She was surprised. We often don't realize how a few small changes each day can make a big difference. Suppose you're hungry between meals and want to grab a quick snack. Here are choices that carry approximately 100 calories each:

1/2 c. fiber cereal like All-Bran with 1/2c. "light" yogurt

3/4 c. blueberries with 1/2c. "light" yogurt

3/4c. strawberries with 1/2c. low-fat cottage cheese

2c. raw vegetables with 2T. low-calorie dressing

3 Finn Crisp crackers and 1T. "light" cream cheese

4c. air-popped popcorn (no added fat)

Here's another way of looking at it: try to "lose" 500 calories every day. Losing 500 calories a day could mean up to 50 pounds lost in one year. Here are some ways to reduce calories:

Instead of regular soda, drink diet soda—135 calories less

Instead of regular yogurt, use "light"—120 calories less

Instead of beer, sparkling water—180 calories less

Instead of pastry, an orange —250 calories less

Instead of a meatball sub with cheese, a turkey sub with mustard— 315 calories less

for the chefs

Here are some ideas for low-fat cooking and eating for the chef in your household. Dr. Tim and I also recommend *Cooking Light Magazine* for healthy, lower fat recipes.

- ✦ Use non-stick pots and pans for foods that require some fat.
- ✦ When you do use fat to cook, use a tablespoon of olive or peanut oil, the beneficial oils.
- ✦ Use chicken broth or tomato juice instead of fat.
- ✦ Use a steamer rack to cook vegetables or fish.
- ✦ Buy lean cuts of meat. Prior to cooking, trim all visible fat. Discard fat that drips from meat.
- ✦ Bake, roast, or broil meats, poultry or fish. Poach poultry or fish in vegetable juice, broth, or seasoned water made from herbs, lemon juice, or wine.
- ✦ Avoid processed meats such as bologna, salami, and hot dogs. Use turkey breast, turkey ham, boiled ham, or lean roast beef.

◆ Generally, the smaller the chicken the leaner it is. When cooking whole chicken, remove the fat from the carcass. Do not eat the skin. When using chicken parts, remove skin before cooking. When making soups, refrigerate the broth and skim the fat from the top.

◆ Select poultry and fish more frequently than red meat. Even the fattiest fish has less saturated fat than the leanest red meat.

◆ Use skim milk. Buy dairy products made from part skim or low-fat milk.

◆ Substitute low-fat or fat-free yogurt for sour cream. To prevent yogurt from separating during cooking, mix one tablespoon cornstarch to eight ounces of yogurt.

◆ Avoid butter. Select margarine that lists liquid vegetable oil as the first ingredient. Or spray "I Can't Believe It's Not Butter," available in a pump, on anything you would put butter on.

◆ Use liquid vegetable oils rich in monounsaturated fats instead of butter, hard margarine, shortening, or lard, which contain saturated fats. Extra-virgin olive oil is best.

◆ Limit total weekly consumption of egg yolks to three, including those used in cooking.

◆ The quality of most baked goods will not suffer if you decrease the amounts of sugar and oil. Experiment. In many cases, pureed fruit can be substituted for most or all of the oil. For the most part, avoid baked goods and pastries.

◆ Commercial salad dressings vary greatly in amount and types of fat. Read the label carefully and buy wisely. Seasoned rice vinegar, lemon, or lime is excellent by itself on salads.

◆ Use beans more often, alone or with small amounts of lean meat.

restaurants: the rules of order

Restaurant eating is a risky business for those of us on special meal plans. Their meals contain fat and sugar that may be hard to detect until the blood sugar test tells the tale. Help yourself avoid "restaurant regret" by choosing a restaurant that offers a wide variety of grilled and roasted foods. Many restaurants support low-fat eating by offering entrees prepared according to American Heart Association guidelines.

Avoid restaurants that offer lots of fried meats and vegetables. Run away from the "all-you-can-eat" brunch. There are too many choices and the temptation to go back one more time is too great. Salad bars also pose a threat to your good intentions. If you stick to fresh vegetables and low-calorie dressings, you'll be fine, but beware of the cheese, chopped eggs, potato salad, gelatins, and high-fat dressings.

Many restaurant meals offer more calories at one sitting than most of us need in a day. If your meal includes an appetizer, avoid the ones that are fried. Try ordering broth soup (no cream) or perhaps pass on the first course. While waiting for your order, be aware of the tendency to fill up on the bread and butter they just plopped down in front of you. If you've calculated a piece of bread into your meal plan, then you'll be fine. If dessert is included, ask for a bowl of fresh berries.

Watch out for hidden fats. Fried foods, cream sauces, gravies, salad dressings, and mayonnaise are the primary culprits. Ask how a dish is prepared. Also asked how it's served. They may roast the turkey and then cover it lavishly with fatty gravy. Order sauces and salad dressings on the side, so you can use only what you need. Of course, you may not be understood. On my first day in Australia, we went to lunch and I ordered a salad. I said, "Please put the dressing on the side." The waitress looked puzzled and then brought my salad. The dressing had been poured onto the plate all around the edges of the greens. I laughed and explained what I had meant. She said, "Oh, you should have asked for your dressing in a jug on the side."

Many restaurants serve huge portions to impress their clientele. When your entrée arrives, eyeball the portions and compare them to the deck of cards image for the protein and the tennis ball image for vegetable and starch servings. If the portions are too large (as they frequently are), you can put some on a side plate and offer a taste to others or ask for a "doggie bag" and take it home for lunch the next day.

Whether you're eating at home or at a restaurant do the best you can to stay on your meal plan. If you ordered your salad with dressing on the side and it arrives doing the backstroke in a sea of Creamy Italian, politely send it back. It's your meal, your body and it's okay to expect exactly what you ordered.

You can learn to steer yourself toward beneficial choices. As noted in the beginning of this chapter, there are three basic instructions for a healthy relationship between food and diabetes: eat a variety of healthy foods, be consistent by eating the same amount of food at about the same time each day, and be flexible. If you are able to put these in place in your daily habits, you'll move toward feeding your body's best interests.

It's never too late
to begin being fit.

chapter seven

tote that barge, lift that bale: the joy and challenges of exercising

Starting an exercise program is not easy. Getting up off the couch is not easy. Getting through the initial discomfort and fatigue is not easy. Staying focused and committed is not easy. Finding the time is not easy. I'll tell you what else is not easy. It's not easy losing your health and being dependent on others for the simplest tasks. It's not easy using a wheelchair or a walker. It's not easy losing your home because you're no longer able to take care of yourself. It's not easy lying in a nursing home, waiting, waiting.

My mother lived the last seven and a half years of her life in "not easy" land. Most of her physical problems were the result of lifestyle choices. Many years before her decline began, she attended a yoga class because she had heard it might be beneficial for her high blood pressure. It helped. Her blood pressure was lower and she didn't have to take as much medication. Then she stopped going to class. She told me it "took too much time. It's easier to just take the pill my doctor gave me." The pill only took away the symptoms, but the underlying imbalances that caused her high blood pressure were not corrected. In less than ten years, she developed congestive heart failure.

Mathematically, the last seven and a half years my mom spent disabled are equal to ten percent of her life. That's 1.6 hours of waking time a day. If even a portion of that time had been spent exercising to increase her strength and stamina, there's a good chance she wouldn't have spent so many years disabled.

your new best friend

By the time you finish this chapter, I'm hoping you'll view exercise as your new best friend. What are the attributes of a friend? I immediately think of someone who brings out the good in me and who has my best interest at heart. Exercise definitely brings out the good in my body and is in my best interest.

Regular exercise increases muscle mass and decreases body fat. It brings tone to the muscles, makes us stronger and more flexible, reduces depression and stress, and improves self-esteem. It increases lung capacity, stamina, and endurance, gives more "giddy-up for your get-along," as my father used to say, and it strengthens the heart. Exercise may also provide anti-inflammatory benefits. A study at the University of Pennsylvania showed that the physical force of blood flow could have an effect on inflammation that is associated with clogged arteries. The study's author, Scott L. Diamond, Ph.D., observed, "We found that elevated blood flow—equivalent to walking at a brisk pace— results in the same sort of anti-inflammatory properties normally associated with high doses of steroids."

Especially relevant to you and Type 2 diabetes is that exercise can lower blood sugar levels and increase the body's sensitivity to insulin. Scientists at Harvard University's Joslin Diabetes Center showed that insulin resistance can be reversed in those who have not yet developed full-blown diabetes. This can happen with just thirty minutes of regular exercise each day. If you have Type 2 diabetes, you may even find that a balanced exercise and nutrition program can bring your blood sugar levels back to normal and eliminate the need for medication. Another study showed that people with diabetes who exercise for an hour three times a week (twenty-five to thirty minutes a day) for eight weeks lowered their HbA1c levels by almost one point. A group of researchers found that people who exercised an hour a day for twelve weeks lost an average of sixteen pounds, with no changes in their diet. Losing weight is beneficial to blood sugar control.

Dr. Kenneth Cooper is founder of the Aerobics Center in Dallas, a nationally renowned research and workout center. Part of his research focus has been to prove that there's a direct relationship between aerobic capacity—your ability to take in oxygen and utilize it—and your ability to avoid major diseases. Walking thirty minutes a day cuts a person's risk of dying from heart disease or stroke by fifty percent, and the risk of dying from cancer, injuries, or degenerative disorders by 60, 70, and 80 percent, respectively. Dr. Charles Clark, Jr., former president of the American Diabetes Association, said, "The data supporting the health benefits of physical activity are overwhelming."

Walking 30 minutes a day cuts a person's risk of dying from heart disease or stroke by 50 percent, and the risk of dying from cancer, injuries, or degenerative disorders by 60, 70, and 80 percent, respectively.

If you haven't been active or are going to begin new activities, it's important that you talk with your doctor and/or diabetes educator before you begin. They'll help you decide which exercises are safe for you to do, because certain forms of exercise carry risks for some people with diabetes. For example, if you have proliferative retinopathy (a condition which, untreated, can lead to blindness—I discuss diabetes' effects on the eyes more in Chapter Eleven) and you do jarring aerobic exercise or heavy weightlifting, bleeding of the eyes can occur or the retina can detach. If you have numbness in your feet or cannot feel them, or if your shoes don't fit properly or you exercise for too long a time, foot ulcers or soft tissue and joint injury can occur. For these complications, exercise such as swimming and bike riding are recommended.

Once you have your doctor's okay, choose an activity that interests you and is appropriate for your age and fitness level. You might think of activities that you've enjoyed in the past. If you're going to take a class, talk with the teacher before you begin. The teacher should know that you have diabetes, plus the warning signs of low blood sugar. You should always have some form of sugar with you and your teacher should know where you keep it and exactly what to do if you need assistance.

Let your teacher also know about any limitations or injuries you have. During class, don't feel you have to keep up with everyone else, especially the first few times you attend. Pay attention to how your body is handling this new activity. If your muscles are shaking or you're out of breath, slow down a little. You don't want to do so much that you are excessively sore. You'll be less likely to repeat a class if you find it hard to move two days later. Let your body slowly become accustomed to this new challenge. In a few weeks or months, you'll be surprised at how much strength and stamina you have gained.

Maintaining a fit body requires three exercise elements: cardiovascular work, strength training, and flexibility. In recent years, we've been hearing more and more about the virtues of being active. Not too long ago, thirty minutes a day was recommended. Just recently, I heard that the recommendation has been increased to sixty minutes a day. That may sound unworkable to you if you're a busy person, but there are many ways to create opportunities for movement. Actually, some of the busiest people I know always make time for exercise, because it gives them the stamina and energy to accomplish their very long "to-do" list.

inspired by an expert

Sheila Cluff is one of those busy people. She is the owner of two popular health spas in California, The Oaks at Ojai, and The Palms at Palm Springs. Sheila began what she calls her "wonderful journey in the world of wellness," in 1959 as a PE teacher in a high school in Canada. She quickly saw that her girls were bored with traditional physical education and came up with abundant excuses to avoid PE. She told me, "I had girls who tried to convince me they had their period every week!" She came up with the idea of adding music to some dance moves and the girls stopped bringing in excuses and started participating. That's when she realized that the key to fitness was making it fun, as she says, "something you want to do, not have to do."

I've known Sheila for almost thirty years. My guess is that she's in her late sixties and yet she leaves all of us trailing behind her on the "brisk walk" she leads through Ojai each morning. She also demonstrates forty pushups at the morning "Mind/Body Awareness" class. Most of the rest of us poop out between ten and twenty pushups.

Sheila has definitely learned how to make fitness fun. My sister, Peggy, and I meet at The Oaks every January for four or five days. We eat delicious spa meals, lose a little weight, and attend many of the fourteen classes offered each day. The classes range from Qi Gong and yoga to belly dancing and water aerobics. I come home really excited and motivated about fitness.

Sheila says, "My team involves our clients in making a lifestyle change so that when they go back to their own world, they're not just fitting fitness in like a prescription which they do for a short period of time. We want to give them the knowledge, the interest, and the motivation to enhance their health, their wealth, and their ability to function effectively. We help them become what we call an activity-oriented person, so they think in terms of movement in the way they live their lives, not movement as an exception."

When it comes to fitness, Sheila believes that body fat percentage is a more important indicator of health and fitness than your weight. She told me, "Being skinny does not necessarily mean you are fit. I had a woman at The Oaks who was anorexic. You could see her bones sticking out all over, and yet she had 40 percent body fat. She had very little lean muscle mass. A woman should be between 21 and 23 percent body fat. We have proven that if you're over 23 percent body fat, you dramatically increase your risk of breast cancer, colon cancer, diabetes, and cervical cancer."

Sheila never asks a woman if she wants to lose weight. She asks if she knows her percentage of body fat. "We tell our clients to go home and throw the scale away." She recommends that you get a tight pair of pants that are a realistic size for you to be, and either grow into them or never grow out of them. Sheila believes that your measurements count more than your weight. Lean muscle takes up less space and weighs more than a comparative volume of fat. Therefore, you can be building muscle and you may not see your weight change by much, but you're losing inches as you replace fat with lean muscle. Lean muscle also burns more sugar than fat does, so having more lean muscle increases your resting metabolism. The higher your aerobic capacity, the higher your metabolic rate. You can check with your diabetes educator or doctor about getting your body fat measured. Your local gym may be able to do it. It's a good predictor of overall health, along with blood pressure, cholesterol, triglycerides, etc.

Sheila feels that fitness is an important key to a happy, healthy life and she walks her talk. She told me, "In the morning, my personal routine is to get up and spend six minutes in yoga postures to loosen up the body. I then do forty pushups, thirty woman's pushups with my knees on the ground, then ten men's pushups. Then I do a series of abdominal exercises, because I've had four children and that's a weak area in our family. Then I do arm work with ten-pound weights. That takes thirty minutes. Then I do my forty minutes of aerobics."

She also recommends what she calls "fitness snacks." For example, while you're waiting for the light to turn to green, or waiting for an elevator or are at security at the airport, stand on one foot and balance. If you're waiting at the doctor's office, practice your balance or stretch a little. If you're worried about looking silly, go out in the hall. At the computer, after an hour or so, get up and stretch to release tension in the neck and back. She wants us all to become what she calls "an activity-oriented person." If you're doing formal training three days a week, then make time for movement on the other days.

She says, "Walk the dog with your grandkids, do some gardening. Do you live in an apartment with stairs? Are there stairs at work you could take even for a few flights instead of the elevator? Just try to do sixty minutes of movement each day."

There are so many benefits to fitness. One of them is a natural "high," and you don't need to go to Colorado to get it. When you work out aerobically, your brain produces a chemical called an endorphin, a cross between a tranquilizer and a stimulator. Exercise also raises your serotonin levels. Low levels of serotonin are noted in depressed individuals and it's the reason drugs like Prozac are prescribed.

Sheila notes, "An aerobic workout that makes you sweat and increases your pulse rate for a minimum of twenty minutes actually has an impact on the appetite. It helps prevent uncontrollable cravings. That stabilization helps people make better food choices. Also as we go through passages in life, especially as women, we tend to be subject to osteoporosis, softening of the bones. We know that weight-bearing exercise, such as lifting weights, walking, and hiking, is an antidote to bone loss. Research is on the cusp of proving that if we take someone with osteoporosis and put them on a weight-bearing program for say six months, we actually can make bones grow again. It's not totally proven yet, but the research is pointing in that direction."

Sheila tells the story of a woman who came to The Oaks who didn't tell them that she had Type 2 diabetes. She checked in with the nurse, but only for her weight and measurements. About five days later, she came back to the nurse and said, "I feel so great, I've taken myself off medication." The nurse asked what medication. She answered, "Oh, I'm a diabetic."

Sheila says, "Of course, we panicked, but we worked with her carefully. She stayed for a month and lost a high percentage of body fat. And do you know that she never had to go back on her medication? She made the necessary lifestyle changes and now comes back twice a year to keep herself motivated."

Sheila wants for you what Dr. Tim and I want. We want you to focus on fitness, health, and good dining in a reasonable manner. You can design a plan that fits your life. Sheila suggests, "You can walk the dog four times a week for thirty minutes. You can keep a set of weights by the kitchen sink and do a little strength training while the coffee is brewing." If you're financially able, you can hire a personal trainer two or three times a week. Whatever method you use, whatever your economic level, being consistent and seeing results is a gift you will give yourself and your loved ones.

on your mark, get set, go!

Okay, now that Sheila's got your attention, let's get started with the basics. If you're going to begin by concentrating on only one form of exercise, it should be a cardiovascular one. It could be walking, swimming, biking outdoors or on a stationary bike, running, rollerblading, dancing, or kickboxing. Current recommendations are that you:

- ✦ Exercise for a minimum of thirty minutes, either in two fifteen-minute sessions or one thirty-minute session.
- ✦ Exercise a minimum of three days a week, building up to five days.
- ✦ Warm up for five to ten minutes and cool down for five to ten minutes, including some stretching after your workout.

Be certain that you have the proper equipment. Choose comfortable, loose-fitting clothing that's right for the activity and the weather, so you can avoid getting too hot or too cold. Wear socks that draw moisture away from your feet. (You can buy them online at www.medicool.com.) Foot powder can also help keep feet dry. Wear comfortable, well-fitting leather shoes that are made for that activity. They should have broad toes and padded heels to help prevent blisters. You might ask your healthcare professional to recommend a store with expertise in fitting shoes. The seams should not be rough and the soles should absorb shock. Each time you put your shoes on, check for lumps, sand, or worn areas that might cause irritation.

If you're walking or running outdoors, take what you may need with you. Carry an emergency food source in case of low blood sugar. Stay hydrated. Drink water before, during, and after exercise to make up for loss from perspiration. Carry a drink with you, or plan rest stops where you can get a drink of water.

Be sure to wear identification showing that you have diabetes. Carry your cell phone or change for a phone call. If you exercise with someone else, tell the person that you have diabetes and describe the symptoms and treatment for low blood sugar in case it happens to you. If possible, exercise 1–2 hours after a meal and be sure to test your blood sugar just before you begin.

warm-up

If you're walking, warm up by walking slowly for the first five minutes, then increase your pace. You can also use the following warm-up:

- ✦ Inhale, lifting your arms overhead, then exhale as the arms return to your sides. Do that 5 or 6 more times.

✦ Alternating, gently lift each knee to your chest 8 to 10 times. Stand near a wall or fence in case you need to steady yourself.

✦ Then tap each foot 15 or 20 times. Then rotate your toes in wide circles to warm the ankles.

If you're weight training, spend five minutes or more on the treadmill first. Your warm-up period gets your heart and muscles ready for harder work. Warm-ups slowly increase your heart rate and loosen up muscles and ligaments, helping prevent dizziness and injury.

intensity

Many activities can be done at a light (leisurely) pace, a moderate pace, which offers aerobic benefits, or an intense (competitive) pace. To increase aerobic fitness, burn fat, and bestow cardiovascular benefits, your intensity needs to be in the moderate range. Research published in *Circulation* magazine reported that men with Type 2 who walked briskly for four hours a week had a lower risk of cardiovascular disease than those who walked at a casual pace did.

Begin your exercise program gently, working to get your heart rate up into its target heart rate, at least 70 percent of maximum. Then, over a period of days, weeks, and months gradually increase your pace. For example, you may start with slow-paced walking the first week or two, and gradually move into brisk walking. Whatever your activity, try to exercise your whole body. For example, swing your arms broadly when walking to exercise your upper body as well as your legs. Keep your back straight and your gaze ahead of you, not down at the street. Breathe deeply. As long as you can still talk to the person next to you, you are working at an appropriate level of intensity. If you are so out of breath that you can't carry on a short conversation, ease up a bit.

If your doctor approves, gradually work up to an aerobic level of activity, which is 80 percent of your maximum heart rate. This pace offers benefits that can increase your heart and lung capacities. A more intense pace is also aerobic, but offers no more benefits than a moderate pace.

your target heart rate

You can ask your doctor, exercise specialist, or diabetes educator to figure out your target heart rate, the heartbeats per minute that are 70 percent to 80 percent of your maximum heart rate for your age and fitness level. It's at this 70 to 80 percent of maximum heart rate that your body will be in the "fat-burning" and "cardio-training" zone. Or you can use the following formula:

> 220—your age = estimated maximum heart rate
> Multiply that by 70 percent and then by 80 percent =
> That's your target heart rate

> For example, if you're 50:
> 220—50 = 170 is your maximum heart rate
> 170 x .70 = 119
> 170 x .80 = 136

So, at 50, your target heart range would be between 119 beats and 136 beats per minute (BPM). The less fit you are, the more quickly you'll get to your target range. As you become more aerobically fit, you'll find yourself having to work a little harder to reach that same target.

You can purchase a small battery-powered heart monitor to give you a constant heart rate readout. After returning from The Oaks, I decided to work on my aerobic fitness and got a heart rate monitor made by Polar that includes a wrist receiver and a transmitter that I wear mid-chest. They have several different models that range in cost from $80 upward. According to my Polar, my target range is 114 to 139. This morning I rode my stationary bike until I was at 125 BPM and then stayed close to that for the rest of my workout.

Or use the low-tech way to compute your heart rate. Pause during exercise, perhaps when you begin to feel just a little out of breath. Using a watch with a second hand, take your pulse for ten seconds. Multiply that by six to approximate your beats per minute. Exercising in your target heart range is the basis of the "New PE," a new approach to school-based physical education that is gaining acceptance across the nation.

duration

When you first begin your exercise program, you may feel like exercising only 5-10 minutes, with 1-2 minutes of warm-up and 1-2 minutes cool-down. (My first day on the stationary bike, I got to eleven minutes and that was it.) As you become fit, you'll build stamina and be able to work out for longer periods of time. (Only five days later, I spent twenty minutes in my target range and I was still feeling pretty good.) For a moderate aerobic program, you will need to work out for a minimum of 15-20 minutes at your target heart rate. Warm-up and cool-down will last about 5-10 minutes each. For weight loss, you need to increase the length of time you exercise, rather than how hard you exercise.

Stop exercising immediately if you have chest pain or severe pain or muscle strain. If you feel lightheaded, faint, or sick to your stomach or think your blood pressure may be getting high, stop. If you're walking or running, slow your pace if you feel really out of breath or before you feel exhausted. Give yourself the "Talk Test" by listening to yourself talk. If heavy breathing interrupts your speech, it's time to slow down. Of course, if you have any signs of low blood sugar, stop and treat it.

Be consistent with your exercise, its intensity, duration, and frequency. By being consistent, your heart and body will be prepared for gradual increases.

cool-down

Slow down your activity before stopping. Your cool-down can be slow walking, or stretching, flexing and rotation exercise, similar to your warm-up. Cool-down allows your heart rate gradually to slow down to its normal rate.

After exercise, test your blood sugar. Testing will tell you if you need to increase or decrease your snacks next time. If needed, eat a snack after a workout to help prevent low blood sugar.

Then, take off your shoes and socks, and carefully inspect your feet. Look for blisters, splinters, or rubbed places. People with diabetes can get skin infections easily, so take care of any irritation immediately. If you see red areas, check your shoes—is there a seam rubbing? Should the shoe be stretched in that area? Do you need different leather shoes? Call your doctor or podiatrist if you have a blister or broken skin that has not started to heal by the next day.

exercise and your blood sugar

Exercising takes sugar out of the bloodstream while you're doing it and boosts your metabolism for several hours afterwards. For this reason, you want to learn how to keep close track of your blood sugar during and after an exercise session. Check your blood sugar level before you begin an exercise session. If it is less than 80 mg/dl, eat 30–45 grams of a quick-acting carbohydrate such as fruit juice, regular soda, raisins, or hard candy. Then follow that with a snack containing protein and complex carbohydrates. Snacks eaten 15–30 minutes before exercise can prevent low blood sugar when you exercise for less than 45 minutes.

The more strenuously you exercise, the larger your snack should be. Be sure you have sugar-containing snacks with you at all times. During sustained exercise of over one hour, eat 15–30 grams of short-acting carbohydrate for every additional 30 minutes of exercise. People who exercise longer than two hours need to either reduce the amount of insulin or continually supplement with carbohydrates as noted above.

Do not inject Regular insulin into any areas that you will be using during your workout. For instance, if you plan to run, don't inject into your thighs. The abdomen is usually the best site for most exercise regimens.

Test your blood sugar after exercise. Because muscles continue to remove sugar from the blood for many hours after activity, you might want to test an hour or so later. Depending on your blood sugar levels, you may need to eat a snack. Test frequently and be alert for symptoms of low blood sugar. Also, test at bedtime and increase your bedtime snack if your blood sugar is low.

Exercising before bedtime places you at greater risk for low blood sugar. Morning is the best time for a workout, but any time is better than none. If you exercise in the evening, be sure to test your blood before bedtime.

✦ ✦ ✦

Your diabetes medication may need adjusting if you have frequent low blood sugar episodes during or after exercise. Work with your doctor or educator to make the necessary adjustments. However, never fail to take your insulin or diabetes pills unless instructed not to do so by your physician.

A word of caution: If you are in poor control, short bursts of intense exercise actually may raise your blood sugar. When combined with insufficient insulin levels, intense exercise increases the release of hormones such as epinephrine that stimulates the production of sugar by the liver. The result is higher than normal blood sugar.

staying the course

I may be wrong, but I don't think getting started is the biggest problem for most of us. I know you can get to one exercise class or take a walk on your lunch hour once in a while. It's staying with it that's the challenge. As the lyric of a song I wrote says, "Though intentions are true, how easily they slip from our view." Exercise takes time and Heaven knows there are so many other things to do! Some of us need to trick ourselves into staying with it. The key is finding a form of exercise that interests you and matches your personality. Then comes the task of putting it on "project status," as Dr. Phil says. People who stay with their fitness regimen plan activity into their day and respect their appointment with fitness as they do their other commitments.

The next step is being committed to a long-term program. What kind of person are you? Are you a person who values reason and intellectual pursuits? The key for you might be gathering information about the benefits of exercise and posting it where you can see it every day.

Are you a visually oriented person? Gather some magazines and cut out pictures of healthy, active people, pictures of what you feel the benefits of a strong, healthy body will look like. Yes, put that grade school student inside to work, choosing images that inspire you and pasting them on brightly colored construction paper to create a collage.

Do you take pride in individual achievement? A goal-oriented activity like tae kwon do or karate might be right for you. You can celebrate your progress when you achieve the next level belt.

If you're a person of faith, you can use your spiritual understanding to appeal for support and guidance. The Bible tells us that the body is the temple of God. Wow. Ask yourself, "How would I treat this body if I really accepted and experienced it as a temple for the Lord?"

Are you a busy mother who works outside the home? My sister gets up half an hour earlier than the rest of her family and goes for a walk before she leaves for the office. Weekends include walks with her children at her side riding their bikes or family hikes on a nearby trail.

Is it difficult for you to motivate yourself? Is there a friend or neighbor who walks in the morning or evening? Perhaps you could walk with them, even part of the way. How about a dance class with your spouse? How about using the delayed-satisfaction ploy your mother used? "You can't watch television until you finish your homework." You could use, "I can't watch *Oprah* until I've gone for my afternoon walk," or some other reward after your exercise sessions.

If you find yourself slacking off a bit, use your imagination to envision what you want your later years to look like. At a diabetes conference, an older man approached and told me proudly that he'd had diabetes for forty-three years. He looked great—slim, muscular, and fit. He said, "I spend one hour at the gym every morning. I never miss. And I have no complications." That's a statement any person with diabetes would like to make.

By the way, laughter is good for your diabetes. Think of it as jogging for your insides. It's been shown to lower blood pressure, rev up the immune system, and release "feel-good" endorphins. Researchers in Japan recently discovered that patients with Type 2 diabetes had a smaller rise in blood sugar if they giggled after a meal. An article in *Diabetes Care* reported that researchers gave participants identical meals on two separate days. Some subjects listened to a dull lecture. Others watched a comedy. Post-meal glucose levels were significantly lower after laughter than after a lecture.

variety is the spice

Just as you wouldn't want to eat exactly the same food every day without variation, the same old exercise program day after day may get boring, both to your body and your mind. You may reach a plateau where your current regimen will seem easy and maybe even hardly worth the effort. You can use your target heart rate to keep yourself working at appropriate levels, and you can begin to vary the frequency and duration of your walks to build more stamina. Shake it up a little. If you're walking three days a week on the treadmill, add an outdoor hike. Ask a little more of your body, paying attention to target heart rate and the "Talk Test." The body possesses a brilliant system of supply and demand. The more you ask of it, the more it works to provide. If you ask for more muscle by weight training, it builds more muscle. If you ask for more lung capacity by breathing more deeply and aerobically than usual, the body lets those new levels become the norm. And it's never too late.

Wilda came to my yoga class as a seventy-eight-year-old high-risk cardiac patient. She was determined to grow stronger and healthier. Because I couldn't give her the one-to-one attention she deserved within a crowded class structure, I sent her to my friend Lauren who teaches Pilates. After her first hour-long session, she went home and fell asleep for two hours in her recliner. But she kept coming back for more. Two years later, Wilda's doctors are amazed. She's off almost all of her medications and is no longer a high-risk cardiac patient. Recently she went to see her doctor and he told her, "Go home. You're too healthy to be here."

Now Wilda walks thirty minutes on her treadmill everyday without being out of breath. She's lost two dress sizes. She feels and looks great and says she's ready to give yoga a try. She told me that when she and her daughters go for a walk, she has to wait for them to catch up. At eighty years old, she's an inspiration to all of us who know her.

Jan is another good example of how to get started and stay with it. She's a patient of Dr. Tim's, fifty years old and has had Type 2 diabetes for ten years. She's been taking oral medications and had gained a lot of weight in recent years. Finally she saw pictures of herself with her family and decided that she looked awful. That did it! She decided she was going to exercise.

Jan set a big goal for herself: to train for a triathlon. When she tried to run, she had pain in her ankles and knees. She talked with Dr. Tim and decided to start slowly with a daily walking program. She worked up to walking four miles in the morning and four miles in the afternoon. Over the course of the next twelve months, she lost fifty pounds. Once the weight came off, she was able to run without any joint pain. She celebrated by buying herself a new bike. Now that she isn't embarrassed to be seen in a bathing suit, she has added swimming.

Jan admits having a hard time staying motivated. When she gets discouraged, she calls friends who also have Type 2 diabetes and they walk and talk together. Or she'll buy new hiking shoes or set a goal for a new adventure. She's so excited about her body's strength and ability that now she's trying new sports: mountain climbing, snowshoeing, and weight-lifting, along with her triathlon training.

It's never too late to begin being fit. Research has shown that fitness can improve into the eighties, nineties, and beyond. After retiring and being diagnosed with diabetes, one woman started exercising with the help of a personal trainer (a gift from her daughters.) She dropped 30 extra pounds, greatly improved the efficiency of her heart, lungs, and circulatory system, and increased her strength and flexibility. Her balance also improved significantly. Falls are a major cause of injury and death in the elderly, so as we grow older maintaining good balance is important.

*. . . we have time to
influence their behavior.
. . . Our children learn
what we teach.*

chapter eight

teach the children well

Parenting is one of the most demanding and difficult jobs any of us will ever have. It's also a job for which we receive no formal training. The challenge of parenting is heightened when diabetes enters the picture. If your child has Type 2 diabetes, she or he is most likely an early or middle teenager who is significantly overweight. Up to 15-20% of America's teens, 12-18 years of age are overweight and obesity is the cause of our epidemic of Type 2 diabetes in children.

We know that too much weight increases insulin resistance, which for many people results in diabetes. There are several factors that cause a child to be overweight and to get diabetes. There may be a history of Type 2 diabetes in the family and genetic factors can also play a role in weight gain. Children whose family members are overweight may have an increased tendency to become overweight. Yet the most important factor concerning weight gain inherited from your family is lifestyle: shared eating and activity habits.

So the bad news is that your child has Type 2 diabetes. The good news is that the circumstances that led to overweight and insulin resistance—too many calories coupled with insufficient exercise—are ones that you and your child can change.

what can i do?

You are your child's first and most important role model. Your first responsibility is to learn everything you can about diabetes and your child's care routine. By doing that, you will be signaling to your child that you care about his or her health and that it's important to pay attention to his or her diabetes.

Along with supporting your child's blood sugar control efforts, you can work with your health care professional to formulate a balanced eating plan that works for the whole family. There are dozens of good cookbooks that will be helpful. Have a wide variety of healthy foods in the house. I always had dried and fresh fruit sitting on the kitchen counter for my kids after school. Microwave low-fat popcorn, lower-fat cheeses like string cheese, raw vegetable sticks and low-fat ranch dressing, and low-sugar yogurt also provide healthy snacks for children with diabetes. Also, make a rule that there's no eating in front of the TV.

Take the time for family meals. Involve your children in shopping for and preparing meals. I got a lot of support for this by instituting the "Hurray" strategy. Each night one of my sons helped me prepare dinner and before we ate, we'd cheer, "One, two, three—Hurray for the chefs!" I didn't want them to think meals magically appeared from nowhere and also wanted them to know how to feed themselves. We still say "Hurray for the chefs" before every meal we eat together.

Make an effort to connect with other parents who have a teen with Type 2 diabetes to share your successes and failures. I know from my own experience that what helped me most was talking to others parents. When Brennan was first diagnosed, I was so overwhelmed that I couldn't possibly retain everything I'd been taught at the hospital, yet I was expected to begin a whole new way of life in just a few days. I really needed someone who understood my fear and frustration. No one understands what you're going through better than another parent of a diabetic teen who's had it for a few years and has already covered some of the ground you're about to traverse. You can use a buddy, believe me.

✦ ✦ ✦

how you can help your child

Your child is going to have some strong feelings about diabetes and its requirements. There are many strategies you can use to help her through this experience.

✦ Be a constant source of support. Let her know she is not alone in this challenge, that you will be at her side every step of the way. Your child needs a safe sounding board. She needs to know she can tell you when she's frustrated, angry, and fed up with caring for her diabetes. You may not to be able to solve that problem for her, but she needs to know you will listen. With a chronic illness like diabetes, feelings build up like steam in a teakettle, and talking about it helps release some of the pressure.

✦ Help educate your child. Your child needs to know what diabetes is and how she can control it. She needs to understand why her blood tests are important, both the daily ones and the HBA1c. She should understand how the foods she eats affect her blood sugar and how to adjust her food, exercise, and medication to keep herself in target range.

Your child also needs to know about the bad news: that diabetes can cause devastating complications. Share the good news, too: that Type 2 diabetes can be reversed in many people by returning to normal weight and appropriate fitness levels.

✦ Share responsibility. Depending on her age, your child may want to take full control of her care from the beginning. My suggestion would be that as long as she is living at home, she should at least share her test results and discuss how things are going with you on a weekly basis. There needs to be someone watching, caring enough to ask questions.

✦ Present a unified influence as parents. If you and your spouse differ on aspects of care, discuss it in private. Talk about disagreements over aspects of her care with her doctor or diabetes educator.

✦ Involve the whole family. You don't want your child to feel like "odd man out" because she has diabetes. From the day Brennan was diagnosed, we all ate the same healthy meals. As you implement the lifestyle changes that diabetes brings, other family members will be impacted. Having all the family members committed to those changes helps everyone develop healthier eating and exercise habits at the same time that you care for your child with diabetes.

The family member with diabetes will be getting much more attention than usual, so the family balance may change. I remember Brennan's little brother, Robin, coming to me when he was four.

He asked, "Mommy, Brennan has diabetes, right?"

"Yes," I answered.

"What do I have?" he asked.

I thought for a moment. "You have cute buns." He smiled and walked away, satisfied.

✦ Increase your family's activity level. The average American child now watches 24 hours of television a week. That's 24 hours that used to be spent in creative or active play. I have a few friends that have taken their televisions out of their homes. They are very happy they did. (And this from a woman who made her living on television.) They told me there's much more family interaction and togetherness. My sister came up with another solution: "T" days. The days of the week that have a "T" in them—Tuesday, Thursday, Saturday— are the only days her family watches TV. Dr. Tim recommends rewarding physical activity with time at the computer or playing video games. Plan activities you can enjoy together. You might take a walk after dinner to talk over the day's events. Or put on some music and have a "dance night." Weekends can be for hiking and biking. Make activity a family priority and your children will follow your lead.

✦ Walk your talk. Follow the advice you give and set an example. Whether it's eating healthy foods or making exercise a priority, you have very little leverage if you're giving advice you're not living.

✦ Talk your walk. Be honest when you're scared or hurt by your child's actions. Don't pretend everything is fine. If your feelings are so inflamed that you feel you might lose control, take a few deep breaths, go for a walk, or call a friend. When you've settled down, sit down with your teen and use "I" messages: "I really feel frightened by your behavior this week." Accusations and blame hinder, not help communication. As my friend Troy says, "Step away from the blamethrower!" Let your teen know that you are worried and upset because you love her and don't want anything to hurt her or limit her life. If things should get to the "non-compliance" stage, get professional help right away. It's your child's health and life that's at risk.

While our teens are still living at home, we have time to influence their behavior. Think of the habits your home life is encouraging. What kind of example are you setting? Our children learn what we teach.

where to turn for support

Primary care physicians rarely have the time or staff to fully address the needs of overweight children with diabetes. They know from experience that telling children and parents to cut back on calories and get more exercise rarely generates results. Because of the long-term danger of obesity and Type 2 diabetes in children, some medical professionals are implementing weight management programs at their local hospitals.

The Weight Management Program at Children's Hospital of the King's Daughters (CHKD) of Norfolk, Virginia is a seven-week course that began in 2001 and now receives referrals from all over the state. They've put together a team that consists of a nurse, a dietitian, a licensed clinical social worker, and a physical therapist. They begin by assessing the family lifestyle and then design weekly homework assignments. They help the parents and child set realistic goals, letting them take baby steps toward losing weight. They try to empower the child to make healthy choices, so parents don't have to constantly act as "food police." Parents learn how to plan meals ahead of time and shop from a list, focusing on fresh foods. They're taught how to read labels on packaged foods. The social worker also plays an important role, because children may overeat for reasons—boredom, anger and sadness—that have nothing to do with hunger. They also hold weekly support meetings. There might be a similar program at your local hospital, staffed by a variety of health professionals, that focuses on behavioral changes for the whole family.

Some family physicians do provide specialized diabetes care. Dr. Tim treats hundreds of adults and some children with Type 2 who are significantly overweight. He has a diabetes educator on staff who works one-to-one with each teen for ten to twenty hours. He's seen that there is a moment in the diabetes education process when a shift occurs.

He says, "It happens at a different point for each person, but it involves a sudden realization, 'This is my problem, not my parents' problem!' Then they begin to do something about it. They exercise and eat properly, and everything changes. They have some success and their self-image improves. They don't all get their weight back to normal, but some lose thirty to forty pounds. They look and feel better. They have to buy new clothes. Their friends comment on the improvement and that encourages them to keep up the effort."

Dr. Gray has made an arrangement with the exercise center next door. As an incentive, he offers his Type 2 clients free use of the equipment if their blood sugar is in good control. Yet the most effective encouragement comes from having active parents and friends. Dr. Tim knows that if everyone around a diabetic teen is a coach potato, it's going to be pretty difficult to get her to break the mold. He told me, "It's tough to get the child to do something if her parents and friends don't."

If teens don't make an appointment as prescribed by their treatment regimen, Dr. Tim sends a letter letting them know it's time to come in. Because they're persistent, Dr. Tim and his staff are usually successful in getting the teens to control their weight and their diabetes.

it's nice to have a friend who has diabetes

When Brennan was twelve years old, he had a close friend, Chris, who also had diabetes. I have a vivid memory of the night Chris came with us to an Italian restaurant. We ordered dinner, and then Brennan and Chris went to the restroom to test blood sugars and give injections.

The boys returned several minutes later, and as they settled into their seats, Brennan looked at me and said, "It's nice to have a friend with diabetes."

Yes, it is. Deborah recently had a chance to be that kind of friend.

Deborah met Wesley when she was substitute teaching, before he had diabetes. A few weeks later, Deborah's friend was the chaperone for a school field trip and she noticed that Wesley had the symptoms of diabetes—excessive thirst and excessive urination. She told his parents to take him to the hospital immediately and indeed, he did have diabetes. Then she put Wesley's parents in touch with Deborah.

Deborah went to visit Wesley in the hospital. She told him they had two things in common: they both have diabetes and they both got it on their ninth birthday. He seemed pretty impressed by that. She also spent time with his parents, telling them not to get discouraged. She said, "Try to stay focused on having him feel good each day. It's like doing a long-term experiment. Some days everything goes just right and some days it doesn't."

Wesley's parents were very encouraged by talking with someone who'd had diabetes for so long who was free from complications. After a few days in the hospital, Wesley went home. Things went well for a week or so and then Deborah got a call. Wesley's parents asked if she would come over and talk with him. He was refusing to do his blood test. He said it hurt too much. As she arrived at his home, she got an idea. Knowing how much Wesley loved soccer, she suggested that pricking his finger was like kicking the soccer ball.

She asked, "When you kick the ball, does it hurt your foot?"

He said, "Yes."

"Have you noticed that the more you kick the ball, the less you think about hurting your foot?"

"Yes."

"And how do you feel when you kick the ball and make the goal?" Deborah asked.

"I feel great. I get excited." Wesley replied.

"Then pretend when you're pricking your finger you're kicking the ball, and once the blood goes into the meter, you've made your goal."

Wesley looked at Deborah and said, "I'm ready to test my blood now."

a diabetes mentor

Most teens are very concerned about being "different." Clinical social worker Beverly Daley, Ph.D. understands what it's like to be a teen with diabetes who's worrying about that issue and she's done something innovative to help.

In 1986, she started a program at Los Angeles Children's Hospital that introduced teens with diabetes to adults who also have it. The first year, ten teenagers paired with ten adult "mentors." The purpose was to provide a relationship with a competent adult who understands the emotional pain of living with diabetes.

Beverly told me, "Many teens are really frightened by diabetes, yet they don't discuss their fears. That makes it difficult to win their cooperation. In spite of their defiance toward parents and medical staff, I've seen that teenagers need adults and they really want to be connected."

The role of the mentor is to be there as a confidant and role model. The emphasis is not on changing behavior; it's on the relationship. The goal is to help the teenager feel good about herself, so that diabetes is not seen as such an obstacle.

Beverly notes, "A teen with diabetes is thinking things like 'How much do I have to look forward to? Am I going to be well? Is anybody going to want me?' Having an adult sponsor who has resolved these issues gives the teen a reason for hope and optimism. The way we've seen it unfold is that the teenager, with a good mentor, is allowed to grow toward competence. It takes a commitment on both sides to stay with the relationship. As the relationship develops, we've seen that the teen admires the adult and feels better about herself. She sees that diabetes can be managed, and she eventually comes to emulate her mentor."

The adult mentors are in their late twenties and early thirties, mostly professionals. They are matched with a teen on the basis of gender, interests, and geographic area and a little old fashioned intuition. The mentors meet every few months for dinner to discuss the ups and the downs of working with the kids. The teens tend to see the adults as parent figures, so even though they agree to be in the program, they often feel defensive about it and about what they're not doing. There is tension caused by their having to be accountable to another adult. It takes a great deal of sensitivity on the part of the mentor to be patient as the relationship develops. Yet that patience reaps rewards. The formal program lasts just one year, but many teens and sponsors stay friends for a long time.

I spoke with Philip, who's been seeing his sponsor for four years. He told me, "It's nice to have someone to relate to and it gave me a better understanding of ways to manage my diabetes. We didn't talk about diabetes that much, but it was good to talk with someone who knew what kind of things I had to deal with. I learned by observation, because he did things differently than I did."

Beverly recently heard from a former teen participant who's now in her twenties and taking good care of herself. The young woman told Beverly that it was a wonderful experience to have a mentor. She had been paired with a nurse who was married and had a baby boy. She said, "It was so comforting to have a relationship with a woman who had diabetes, who had a husband and a healthy baby, and who wasn't limited by diabetes."

Beverly was pleased to hear such long-term enthusiasm about the program. "The fact that she could say that to me after all these years shows that it was really worth it. It says a great deal about what it means to a young person who is possibly feeling doomed as a result of having diabetes. It's very profound to give them this kind of hope that they are willing to make a commitment to take care of themselves."

Beverly did a study looking at the effect of the program on self-esteem and diabetes care. There was a difference between the control group and those teens that had mentors. The mentored teens were less likely to agree, "I wish I could run away" and "I wish I didn't have diabetes."

A similar program was set up through a school of social work at a hospital in Tel Aviv. Beverly is in frequent communication with them and they've reported a very good outcome with the first ten mentor pairings.

Beverly says, "My sense of the program is that it's a very powerful intervention. The kids really do need this kind of support and they do value it. It does ultimately help them make some kind of commitment to taking better care of themselves."

If you like the idea, talk with your doctor and diabetes educator about locating a diabetes mentor for your child. By the way, while you're at it, locate a parent mentor for yourself.

school daze

No matter how well you implement good eating and exercise habits at home, when your child leaves for school and time with friends, all bets are off. With the addition of fast food and vending machines stocked with soda and candy, along with the deletion of physical education programs, school campuses can be detrimental to the health of our children.

There are other obstacles. Keeping blood-testing equipment at the school is sometimes eyed with suspicion. One mother was told that school officials were worried that the equipment had something to do with drugs and drug abuse. I've heard from parents that they had to put up quite a battle to get their local school board to allow blood tests at school, even under the guidance of a staff person in the school office. If necessary, get a letter from your child's doctor explaining the nature of your child's diabetes care and why the equipment is essential. If you run into trouble, try to be patient. Few people know as much as you and your child do about diabetes. Being able to clearly explain diabetes will help others become more sensitive toward people who have it.

Before you talk with office staff or school personnel, let your child know what you're going to do. Your child may not want anyone to know. That's understandable. You can explain that whether or not her friends know is her business, but someone at school must know what to do in case there's an emergency. Some children decide to be honest about it. I remember hearing of a young boy with Type 1 who presented a science report about diabetes to his class. A classmate remarked, "I had diarrhea once."

Even though seriously low blood sugar in someone with Type 2 is rare, there might be a morning when your teen runs out of the house without having an adequate breakfast. By mid-morning, she might be feeling shaky and nauseous if her blood sugar drops too low. The school's staff needs to know about low blood sugar and how to treat it. Have a clear directive on file at the school office about what to do if your child feels unwell. They should know to do a blood test right away. If the reading is low, they can treat it with juice or sweetened soda (not diet soda.) If the blood sugar is high, have them call you or your child's doctor. Make sure everything is written down and that school personnel know how to reach you during school hours.

Many schools nowadays do not have a nurse on campus and untrained personnel are expected to handle medical situations. One newly diagnosed fourteen year-old client of Dr. Tim's wasn't feeling well and went to the school office. A staff member tested him and his blood sugar was high— 230. He told them it should be 100 to 150. They tested him ten minutes later. Still high. After eleven tests, they finally called his mother. The mother said, "Don't do anything else. I'll come over and write down what you should do so you have it from now on."

You might also want to meet with the cafeteria manager. School lunches are often high in sugar, fat, and salt, although some communities are addressing those issues. It's important for your child to be a child first and a child with diabetes second. She's going to want to be like the other kids. If you can't get her to take a healthy lunch from home, try to get a copy of the school lunch menu a month in advance. The two of you can look through the menu and notice which foods are not going to be "good" for her.

If you have problems getting your child's needs met at school, consult your doctor, a lawyer, or call TASK—Teams of Advocates for Special Kids. They train parents to use legal means to make certain their children are afforded equal education and consideration under the law. Your child's rights are protected under the federal Education of All Handicapped Children's Act which states that all children, handicapped or otherwise, must be provided with the services they need in order to benefit from public education. Section 704 of the Rehabilitation Act also provides protection for people with diabetes, asthma, epilepsy, and other chronic diseases. TASK has a web site at www.taskca.org or call 1-714-533-TASK.

coming of age

Children in their teens undergo rapid physical and psychological changes. These changes make controlling diabetes even more difficult. Just at the time when your teen wants more independence and self-determination, diabetes coupled with hormonal changes makes close medical supervision a must. It's a tough combination.

The teen years span a turbulent time of becoming an individual, separate but equal (so they think) to their parents. Your teen may be at the stage of rejecting your values and rules. I remember the day my normally cuddly Brennan walked into the kitchen with a disapproving look and said, "Why do you wear those big belts?" He was thirteen.

I thought, "So . . . it's begun." It reminded me of a girlfriend telling me of her daughter's thirteenth birthday. My friend walked into the kitchen in the morning and wished her daughter "happy birthday." The daughter burst into tears and ran sobbing from the room. She said, "For the next four years, everything I did was wrong."

Dr. Tim says the tricky part of a teen's mood swings is that you can't always be sure if it's caused by fluctuating hormones or low blood sugar.

In addition to being adamant that they will not be "like you," most teens are also extremely sensitive to "being different." They may skip taking their medication, eat whatever their peers are eating, or stop blood testing just to prove that they are "not different." Before we as parents get in an uproar over this kind of "rebellion," we have to perform a parental reality check. We really can't expect anyone, much less a teen, to always stick to a preplanned diet. When departures occur, blood tests will tell the tale. That's the time to gently ask, "Any idea of what might have caused this?" Then decide how best to bring the blood sugar closer to normal levels. Also discuss what choices might have been better. Emphasize the "can haves," not the "can't haves."

You may notice I don't use the word "cheating." Paul Madden from the Joslin Diabetes Center in Boston recommends that we drop that word from our diabetes vocabulary. He prefers that less judgmental approach, using terms like "overeating" or a phrase like "you ate more than your body needed at the time."

When dealing with a teenager, especially one who lives with diabetes, you need to know how to pick your battles. Some things are really important; some things aren't. At fourteen, Brennan decided he didn't like the natural curl in his hair and wanted to straighten and lighten it. I wasn't crazy about the idea, and asked him if he really thought it was a good idea.

He told me, "Mom, I'm a teenager. It's my job to experiment with how I want to look and what I want to do."

He was right. "Okay," I said, "I'll make you a deal. You can do whatever you want to your hair. Die it magenta if you like. I ask three things: take care of your diabetes, do your homework, and use good manners." He agreed.

There are so many conflicted feelings for a teen. He's still a child and not ready to be alone in the world, yet he's also a blossoming adult who is making more and more of his own decisions. Many times he is absolutely certain that he is right and his parents can't possibly understand him. One father I know dealt with that by putting a sign on the refrigerator that read, "Teenagers! Are you tired of being pushed around by parents and teachers? Fight back! Move out now, while you still know everything!"

Independence is the big issue. Up until the mid-teen years, you may have been able to dictate what your child did and what he ate, but not any longer. By the time Brennan had reached fifteen, he'd had diabetes for eleven years. I'd always been an essential part of each diabetes decision. He turned to me one day and said, "Mom, I can take care of this myself."

As your teen probably sees it, it's his life, not yours and he wants to make decisions about how he lives. The problem can be that, even though a teen may know about the threat of diabetes complications, some don't take them seriously or don't want to think about it. Nagging and threats don't work. Keeping the lines of communication open is vital.

Just at the time your teen is trying to manage his diabetes, his blood sugar may become more difficult to control. Increased hormonal activity can add extra insulin resistance. The menstrual cycle also adds rising hormonal levels that can reduce the effectiveness of medication.

One other note, poor blood sugar control can delay puberty and menstruation. This may cause concern, but be assured, if the hormones and thyroid are normal, the delay will correct itself as soon as a young woman's blood sugar is under control. Blood sugar control can also become more difficult during menstruation, as there can be a rise in blood sugar during the first few days of the monthly flow. One thirteen-year-old with Type 1 who'd just begun her menses had to test her blood sugar eight to ten times a day to help keep it under control.

Teenagers go through a lot of changes in a few years. They need a compassionate shepherd. That's you—someone who will help them stay in green pastures and away from the ever-present dangers of modern life. I can attest from personal experience: to get them through those years safely is an accomplishment. If you're just beginning that journey, try to be patient and maintain your sense of humor. It helps!

. . . no matter how expert you become, there will be occasions when your blood sugar is either too low or too high.

chapter nine

valley low, mountain high

During a concert tour in Australia, my musical director (who has diabetes) had a low blood sugar episode that got me moving. Before we left for Australia, I promised his wife I would watch over him. At the end of the rehearsal for our first concert, Larry asked me to wait a few minutes so he could test his blood sugar before we left for dinner. He came back and said, "It's 60 and I took my shot." Of course, a "60" blood sugar is low and taking insulin lowers blood sugar even more. Yet Larry looked so clear-eyed and confident that I didn't question him. I assumed he'd eaten some glucose tablets backstage before his shot.

We got to the restaurant and ordered dinner. I looked across the table and Larry was trying to unzip his fanny pack where he kept his diabetes supplies. He had hold of the zipper pull, but couldn't seem to move it.

I asked, "Larry, are you all right?" He looked up, eyes glazed and unfocused, hands lying limply in his lap. He couldn't even speak. I jumped up and headed to the bar, "I need a glass of Coke, right now please! It's an emergency." I was panicked that Larry was so far down that he would have a seizure. Luckily, he was able to drink the Coke. In a few minutes his eyes were once again focused. He followed up with dinner and was fine. Larry's blood sugar was already low after rehearsal and he was confused. That's why he took a shot when what he really needed was sugar-containing food or drink to bring him back up to normal levels.

Your main task as a person with diabetes is to try to mimic your body's natural blood sugar control. It is such a demanding task that I think everyone who successfully manages diabetes should receive an "MBSC"—a "Master's of Blood Sugar Control." Yet no matter how expert you become, there will be occasions when your blood sugar is either too low or too high.

low blood sugar

Low blood sugar is called hypoglycemia. "Hypo" means under, beneath, or below. "Glycemia" is derived from the Greek *glykys*, meaning sweet. High blood sugar is called hyperglycemia. "Hyper" is from the Greek *hyper* meaning over or above.

If your blood sugar falls below 60mg/dl, you have low blood sugar or hypoglycemia. There are lots of reasons this happens: perhaps you accidentally overdosed on medication, mistimed your pills or shots, missed a meal or snack, or exercised without compensating with extra food. Most often, you'll be able to tell you're "low" by the way you feel: shaky, nauseous, nervous, irritable, weak, and/or hungry. Each person has a personal set of symptoms. As you become familiar with the way your body manifests low blood sugar, you'll be able to react quickly. If you can still see straight, test your blood sugar to confirm your feeling.

When your blood sugar is low, you must treat it immediately. The glucose in your bloodstream is your brain's energy source. When levels fall far below normal, you can experience confusion, dizziness, blackouts, mental impairment, lethargy, and seizures.

The basic reasons for low blood sugar include too little food, too much exercise, and too much insulin or diabetes medicine. Maybe your meal or snack was delayed, or you skipped a meal. Perhaps you didn't eat enough protein or carbohydrate to balance your insulin or medication.

If you're "low," maybe your activity level is responsible. Were you more active than usual or did you exercise without eating a meal or snack first?

Or perhaps you took more insulin or pills than prescribed. Did you forget that you took your pills and then take them again by mistake? Another contributing factor can be hormonal changes during the first trimester of pregnancy and at the start of a woman's period.

Because low sugar can happen suddenly and be potentially dangerous, *always carry an easily consumed carbohydrate source with you.* It can be hard candies like LifeSavers or a small tube of cake frosting, 1/2 cup fruit juice, half a glass of sugared soda like Sprite or Coke, 2 tablespoons of raisins or a small piece of fruit, a cookie, or commercial glucose gel or tablets.

Wait 10 to 15 minutes and repeat the treatment if your blood sugar is not back up to normal levels—80 to 120. You may need to repeat a third time if your blood sugar was very low. If your next scheduled meal is more than one hour away, you might want to follow up with a protein snack like cheese and crackers, bread and peanut butter, milk and crackers, or half of a sandwich.

It's important for you to record in your daily record, the time, blood sugar reading, symptoms, and food eaten after any incident. Also, educate your friends and family members so they can offer assistance to you if it is needed. Low blood sugar comes on suddenly, so act quickly to correct it.

low blood sugar sensitivity

A consistent diabetes care regimen is your best defense against low blood sugars. If you've had uncontrolled diabetes for a period of time, you may not recognize the warning signs of low blood sugar: fatigue, sleepiness, and the inability to think clearly. Driving a car while you have low blood sugar can lead to accidents. My friend, Jerry, who has had diabetes since before blood testing, didn't like to test his blood sugar and kept reassuring his doctor that he could tell when he was getting low. Then he lost consciousness while driving and almost drove off the side of a mountain. Fortunately, he was not hurt and didn't hurt anyone else. He started testing his blood sugar shortly after that incident.

Another friend, Jerry, was having trouble with undetected low blood sugar. He wouldn't notice any warning signs until his blood sugar had dropped to

40 to 50. He remembers sitting in the doctor's waiting room and feeling dizzy. He tested his blood and it was 37!

I said, "That could be a real problem if you're driving . . . "

Jerry interjected, "Or walking!"

Jerry's doctor told him that his many years of diabetes had destroyed the mechanism that issues warnings about low blood sugar. Yet Larry has since regained the ability to detect low blood sugar before it gets into the dangerous range. Because of improving his overall daily control, he now feels the warning signs at 60 to 70, a twenty-point improvement and well above the dangerous range.

Deborah also was slipping into some very low blood sugar episodes. When she allowed herself to run slightly higher levels for a week or so without any lows, she regained the ability to feel her blood sugar fall below normal range. By the way, her doctor also had told her that because she'd had diabetes for so many years, she'd permanently lost the ability to sense low blood sugar. That's not necessarily true, as both my friends learned.

Deborah and Larry's experience confirms what recent studies have shown. There's a phenomenon in which the early warning signs of hypoglycemia become very subtle, even undetectable, in those who have recently had another low blood sugar. The theory is that when you have a lower than normal blood sugar, the body may "down-regulate," resetting its response to a lower level for the next low blood sugar. This means that the sympathetic nervous system that normally responds to low blood sugar levels of 50 to 70 mg/dl reprograms itself, so that it doesn't kick in until the blood sugar reaches 30 to 50 mg/dl. The good news is that the reprogrammed response may be temporary and can readjust within a few days of normal blood sugar levels. Basically, the fewer low blood sugar incidents you have, the quicker your body lets you know when you are having one.

One more thing: more than 50 percent of all severe incidents of hypo-glycemia happen during the night. Although it's much more likely to be a problem for those of us who take insulin, you should be aware that it could happen. You can protect yourself from nocturnal hypoglycemia by taking your medications and meals on time.

Another effective tool which I mentioned briefly in Chapter Four is the new Glucowatch that reads blood sugar levels through your skin and sounds an alarm if it gets too low. We'll list information on it in the Resources section.

high blood sugar

Hyperglycemia is not as immediately threatening as low blood sugar, but it's not desirable in the least. It's the years of higher than normal blood sugar levels that cause diabetes complications.

The warning signs of high blood sugar are increased thirst, frequent urination, unexplained weight loss, fatigue, blurred vision, poor healing of wounds, dry, itchy skin, and abdominal pains. Sustained hyperglycemia is toxic to the nervous system and causes numbness and tingling. Or you may not experience any symptoms. Whether you do or not, if you are testing your blood sugar each day, you'll catch high blood sugar as it's occurring.

The reasons for high blood sugar include:

1. Too little insulin. Did you skip a dose of diabetes medicine? Did you take less than the prescribed dose? Did you take it earlier or later than usual?
2. Too much food. Were your servings too big? Did you eat too often? Did you eat too much fat? Or carbohydrate? Or protein?
3. Not enough exercise. Did you exercise? Did you do less exercise than you usually do? Did you exercise when blood sugar is above 240 mg/dl? Did you exercise when your blood sugar was too high?
4. Too much stress or anger. Have you been under stress, either good or bad? Did you get angry? Are you in the midst of a major life change?
5. Illness or infection. Are you feeling sick? Is your temperature elevated? Do you possibly have an infection somewhere?

How do you keep high blood sugars to a minimum? Same old, same old: take your diabetes medicine as directed, follow your meal plan. And keep a consistent exercise regimen. (But don't exercise if your blood sugar is over 240 mg/dl or when you're sick.)

If you're taking insulin and all your blood sugars are elevated, try using a new bottle of insulin. Your insulin may have gotten too warm or too cold and stopped working. It may have expired. The same may be true of oral medication. The one you're taking may no longer be sufficient for your body's needs. You will also want to check your blood test strips to be sure they have not expired.

Please don't ignore high blood sugar, because it can lead to serious problems. A high blood sugar level of 800 to 1200 causes the blood to thicken and results in massive fluid loss and severe dehydration. When high blood sugar and dehydration occur together with Type 2 diabetes, they can result in hyperglycemic hyperosmolar nonketotic syndrome or HHNS. Elderly persons with diabetes who fail to drink enough fluids or care for their diabetes properly are most frequently diagnosed with HHNS. Some become so dehydrated their lips stick together. A person with HHNS is highly susceptible to seizures and coma, and should be hospitalized immediately.

sick days

One of the most difficult times to keep your blood sugar under control will be during illness. If it's an illness you're treating at home, such as a cold or flu, you need to understand how it will affect your blood sugar. If you're in the hospital for an emergency or pre-planned surgery, there is additional advice that is essential.

Illness presents a compromise between eating less with decreased insulin needs and the sickness that increases your insulin needs. Any infectious disease puts stress on the body. In response, your body produces hormones, chemical messengers that tell the liver to release stored glucose into the bloodstream. The extra glucose helps give your body a source of energy to fight the illness. These same hormones also make the body's cells more resistant to insulin. If you're already insulin resistant, as in Type 2 diabetes, the extra released glucose stays in your blood and leads to a rise in blood sugar. This sets the stage for extremely high blood sugar levels and ketoacidosis.

Ketoacidosis is a state in which the body is slowly being poisoned. It occurs when there is too much sugar and too little insulin to move the sugar into the cells. Since the body needs fuel to keep going, the body begins to burn its own fat as fuel. This may sound like a good thing— "I'm burning fat. Yippee!" However, when the body burns fat, waste products called ketones build up in the blood. Ketones make the blood more acidic and disturb the body's chemical balance. The body tries to compensate for this chemical imbalance with deep breathing, and then with even more rapid respiration. A person with ketoacidosis may seem to be out of breath. If untreated, this poisoning process leads to abdominal cramps, vomiting, and severe dehydration.

Melodie was a newlywed and had just taken her first teaching position sixty miles from home. She worked long hours to prepare lesson plans and drove many roundtrips to prepare her classroom for the opening of school. She developed a sore throat and felt so sick that she was unable to eat, so she stopped taking her insulin and her normal care routine. Her new husband had no idea what to do for her. When she finally tested her blood, the glucose level was too high to measure and she tested positive for ketones in her urine. She was in a state of ketoacidosis.

Her doctor told her to go straight to the emergency room. Even though she wasn't eating, two days of not taking insulin resulted in blood sugar over 800 and severe dehydration. She was put on an insulin IV and given fluids to rehydrate her. Her blood sugars decreased and she was able to go home and resume her normal care routine. She and her husband attended diabetes classes together to help them both understand her disease better.

Ketoacidosis is a life-threatening emergency that can result in diabetic coma and even death. Prompt medical treatment is essential and usually includes hospitalization with insulin by IV drip, close blood sugar monitoring, and rehydration with IV fluids.

While most incidents of ketoacidosis occur with Type 1 diabetes, it is important to know the symptoms. They include:

✦   Feeling thirstier or hungrier than usual
✦   Having to urinate more frequently

- Losing weight without dieting or increasing your physical activity
- Feeling more tired or sleepy than usual
- Vomiting or feeling sick to your stomach
- Having stomach pain
- Having a fruity smell on your breath
- Breathing fast and deep
- Blood sugar over 240 mg/dl
- Being dehydrated
- Feeling drowsy for no reason

what to do when you are sick

First of all, treat the underlying illness. You may be advised to take an antibiotic for an infection or Tylenol for fever. If your own doctor is not available, be certain the doctor treating you knows you have diabetes. Then:

- Prevent dehydration—Drink one cup (8 oz.) of fluid every 1/2 to 1 hour. Alternate salty and low-salt fluids, such as bouillon and apple juice. If you're able to eat, follow your meal plan and use sugar-free fluids. If you're not able to keep food down, alternate sugar-containing fluids with sugar-free fluids.
- Take your medication. Do not stop your diabetes pills or insulin, even if you can't eat. Check with your doctor to adjust your dosage.
- Check your blood sugar every 2–4 hours. Set an alarm to check during the night or have someone wake you and take your blood sugar. Continue checking as long as your blood sugars are elevated and/or until symptoms of illness disappear.
- When your blood sugar is over 240 mg/dl, test for ketones. Ketone testing strips are available without a prescription. You dip them in a small amount of urine and read the result—low, medium, or high. If you are spilling ketones, call your doctor.
- Rest. Do not exercise as it may increase your blood sugar.
- Take your temperature morning and evening. If your temperature is one-half degree above your normal temperature, drink extra water.

♦ Check your weight every day. If one-half pound or more weight loss is noted per day, drink extra water.

♦ Note your level of alertness every four hours. If you constantly feel sleepy or can't concentrate, have someone call your doctor.

♦ Monitor your fluid intake. Drink at least twelve 8 oz. glasses of water a day. If it won't stay down, call your doctor right away. You may need to go to the hospital.

♦ If your ketones increase from low to medium or from medium to high along with high blood sugar, call your doctor. If you also experience sleepiness, confusion, and nausea or vomiting along with an increase in ketones, call your doctor and then have someone drive you to the hospital emergency room immediately.

♦ If you are alone, ask someone to call you morning and evening. Instruct him or her that if you don't answer the phone, they should come over and check on you. Also, if you're so sick you feel groggy, let them know your insulin or medication needs so they can help you track how much you're taking. Or have a pen and paper next to the bed and write down when you take medication and how much you take. If you're so sick that you don't feel you can do that, have someone stay with you to monitor your condition.

Dr. Tim has seen many medication errors made while someone is groggy from sleep or illness. He says, "We ask our patients not to keep their medications at the bedside unless it's for emergencies. It's safer to get out of bed and go to the bathroom or kitchen to take medication, especially for people who wake up slowly. Once they walk around for a few minutes, they're usually more alert."

what to eat on sick days

If you can't eat your regular foods, replace them with carbohydrates in the form of liquids or soft foods. Eat at least 50 grams of carbohydrates every three to four hours. You can mix or match the following, or one fruit, milk, or bread exchange can be traded for each 15 grams of carbohydrates.

SERVING SIZE	FOOD	GMS CARBOHYDRATES
1/2 cup	Apple juice/apple sauce	15
1/3 cup	Cranberry juice/ grape juice	15
1/2 cup	Orange juice	15
1/2 cup	Regular ginger ale or 7-Up	10
1/3 cup	Grape juice	15
1 twin pop	Popsicle	24
1/2 cup	Regular gelatin	20
1/2 cup	Cooked cereal	15
1 cup	Chicken noodle soup	10
1/2 cup	Ice cream (vanilla)	15
1/2 cup	Sherbet	30
1/2 cup	Instant pudding	30
1/2 cup	Custard	15
1/2 cup	Fruit-flavored yogurt	20
1 cup	Fruit-flavored yogurt (Sweetened with aspartame)	12
6	Saltine crackers	15
1	Slice bread/dry toast	15
3/4 cup	Gatorade	10
1 cup	Tomato soup	12
1 cup	Milk	12

Sick days can be tricky for people with diabetes. It's a good idea to be prepared and have the items listed below in a sturdy, transportable box. Having them all in one place means that you won't have to search for something you desperately need when you least feel like looking for it. In the box, you'll want to have:

✦ Phone numbers for your doctor, diabetes educator, pharmacy, and hospital.

✦ A copy of the two sections in this book, "What to Do When You Are Sick" and "What to Eat on Sick Days"

✦ Ketone test strips (especially for Type 1 diabetes)

✦ Thermometer

✦ Record or log book to record information

✦ Tylenol, throat lozenges, decongestant, cough medicine, Imodium for diarrhea

✦ Anti-nausea medicine (essential for pump users)

✦ A glucagon kit: Glucagon is a hormone that helps raise blood sugar. In the event of a stomach virus, you may find it difficult to keep your blood sugar in the normal range. If you can't keep any food down, you may need to use the glucagon to bring up a very low reading. Your doctor or educator will advise you how to use it and when.

✦ Sick day menu or sick day foods list

✦ Sick day foods you prefer—regular soda, regular Jell-O, bouillon soup, juice, crackers, regular instant pudding.

One last thing: emotional stress causes you to produce cortisol, the stress hormone, and can have can have the same effect on your blood sugar levels as illness. We'll deal with stress in the next chapter.

hospitalization

Whether you have an emergency like a broken leg, needing stitches, or a pre-planned surgery, it's vitally important that all hospital personnel know that you have diabetes. There are some procedures that might be harmful to your diabetes control. It's a good idea to wear a medical bracelet or necklace tag identifying you as having diabetes at all times.

There are a few factors to consider if you're going to have surgery.

✦   Is the surgery really necessary? Did you get a second opinion?

✦   Is the surgeon familiar with diabetes? If not, make certain there is a physician in attendance who is.

✦   What tests and procedures will be done? Get a list in advance and go over them with your diabetes specialist to have a plan for how to control your blood sugar during your hospital stay. Make sure the plan is in your hospital chart and that all the nurses and doctors know about it.

It is wise to have a person who is familiar with your diabetes care with you in the hospital or available by cell phone. Also be certain that your doctor or diabetes educator are on call during your stay. Ask questions about every medication that they give you to be certain it's approved. Hospital staff can make mistakes.

The stress of surgery puts an additional burden on your body. High blood sugar interferes with healing, so keeping your blood sugar in good control is important.

and away we go . . .

Tammi has had Type 1 diabetes for more than ten years. She works in the international business community as an economic development consultant. She's worked in Russia, traveled throughout sub-Saharan Africa, to France, the United Kingdom, Hong Kong, and Beijing. In 1993, not long after she was diagnosed, she spent a year in Nairobi, Kenya. She stocked several months of diabetes supplies and took them with her. Then she made some trips home during that year for R&R and fresh supplies. There were days she was traveling out in the bush on safari or climbing Mt. Kilimanjaro, yet she always managed to keep herself in good control.

When you're traveling your eating patterns will be disrupted, so spend time in advance of your trip with your diabetes educator to discuss how to adjust your food and medication plan. Use that new plan to guide you to select foods during your trip. If mealtime is delayed, you can eat a small amount of fruit or half sandwich to prevent hypoglycemia until you can eat your meal. You can eyeball the food portions and try to avoid foods high in sugar and fat.

With the changes in schedule that travel brings, you will want to be careful to match your food intake and activity level. As a guideline for very active days of hiking or walking, increase your intake of foods high in complex carbohydrates. For lazy, quiet days, decrease your intake. If you take insulin, and know how to adjust it, you may need less Regular or fast-acting insulin on active days and more on days you aren't exercising.

When you travel, your blood sugar levels will be affected, but you still take good care of your diabetes, as Tammi has. It just takes some planning . . .

- *Have a plan from your health professional* concerning how to adjust your medication if you're traveling across time zones.
- *Carry identification* that indicates you have diabetes and what medications you take. Also, *wear a medical alert bracelet* stating your condition (diabetes) and an emergency phone number.
- *Contact your health insurance* to see if they will cover you in an emergency overseas.
- *Learn how to say,* "I need some juice or sugar immediately," "I have diabetes," and "I need a doctor" in the local language. Have the phrases written down and carry them in your wallet.
- Be sure to *take an extra supply of all medications* and testing equipment. Keep them with you enroute, not checked in your luggage. You may have difficulty purchasing the insulin or your other medications at your destination.
- If you're traveling out of the country, *have your doctor write a letter detailing your condition* and explaining any care issues another doctor might need to know. You can research the name of a diabetes doctor who practices in the area you'll be visiting by contacting the American Diabetes Association or for international travel, the International Diabetes Federation (see resources). Once you've arrived, American embassies and consulates can be helpful

or your hotel may have a list of English-speaking doctors. If it's an emergency, go to the nearest hospital.

✦ *Keep prescriptions for your insulin, syringes, and testing equipment in your wallet.* Some states do not allow purchase of syringes without a prescription. Airlines are now requiring proof of a prescription before allowing you to carry syringes, lancets, and insulin on a plane. Call the airline at least one day in advance to secure the exact requirements for air transportation of your supplies.

✦ *Remember that your insulin requires special handling,* as it will not work if it freezes or becomes too warm (above 86 degrees). Carry your insulin with you in an insulated carrying case. None of your diabetes supplies (except extra food) should be in your checked luggage.

✦ When traveling alone on a bus, boat, or airplane, *let the person next to you know that you have diabetes,* in case you need medical attention. Explain what they can do for you if you have low blood sugar symptoms, telling them if you prefer the glucose tablets in your bag or soda or juice. You can also mention your diabetes to the flight attendant, driver, or tour guide.

✦ *Avoid overexposure to the sun.* Sunburn is stressful to the body and can affect blood sugar. Take sunscreen and a hat with you on your trip.

✦ *Don't wear new shoes when you travel!* There's nothing worse than walking all over Paris your first day and limping for the next four. (I know. I've done it.) Bring shoes and socks that will not irritate your feet or legs in any way. If your feet perspire, you may need to change your socks more often than once a day.

hiking

If you're hiking in the mountains or traveling south of the border, consider the safety of the drinking water. Be cautious of contaminated water or raw leafy vegetables and fruits. If in doubt, also avoid the ice cubes. Drink beverages made from boiled water, such as coffee, tea, or bouillon. These precautions are helpful to prevent diarrhea and blood sugar imbalances. Pack Imodium pills (available over the counter) with you on all trips in case you get diarrhea.

When hiking, wear a backpack packed with plenty of food and glucose tablets, water, a space blanket, Band-Aids, sunglasses, sunscreen, topical antibiotic ointment, a tiny flashlight, matches, extra socks, sweater or sweatshirt, and poncho. If you require insulin, you should carry those supplies also. Some people carry a water-purifying tablet in case they are lost and need to drink stream water.

traveling by car

If you are the driver, test your blood sugar before you get behind the wheel and every two hours while you are driving. Be sure you have eaten adequately to prevent low blood sugar. Don't skip any meals or snacks.

Pull off the road immediately if you feel drowsy or sick. Have emergency food in your car so you can reach it—things like LifeSavers, glucose tablets, a can of juice or regular pop, or fifteen raisins. Once you eat the emergency food, wait 10–15 minutes, then when you feel better, eat follow-up food such as a package of crackers and cheese or crackers and peanut butter.

Bring along extra food for a planned stop or an unexpected delay such as car trouble. You should have an emergency box in your trunk at all times with enough supplies to last you for twenty-four hours, a gallon of water and spare blanket for each person in the car.

Stop for a short break every 1 1/2 hours or so and take a short walk.

bus, train, or boat

Be prepared with snacks or a sandwich. If you are traveling alone, inform the driver, conductor, or cruise director that you have diabetes just in case you have a problem.

Since special meals may be available on a cruise, inquire when you make you reservations and when you first get onboard.

Take motion-sickness medicine with you as well as your extra sources of food.

airplane travel

When you make your airline reservations, ask about special meals available. You can order a diabetic meal, vegetarian meal, or low-cholesterol meal. Confirm the special meal twenty-four hours before your flight time.

Bring emergency foods such as dried fruit, cookies and crackers, and cheese in your carry-on bag. Drink a lot of water before and during your flight to prevent dehydration.

Book an aisle seat ahead of time so you can get up and move around to prevent blood clots and thrombophlebitis in your legs. There have been reports of deaths from these conditions after long airplane flights. Walk up and down the aisles every hour or so to stimulate your circulation.

immunizations

A flu vaccine is recommended yearly for all persons who have diabetes. Ask your doctor when the vaccines are available.

Pneumonia vaccine is available. You should also discuss this with your doctor, as it is recommended for persons who have diabetes. The vaccine provides long-term protection for most people. However, some people may lose protection about six years after vaccination.

Tetanus vaccine is usually administered as a booster every ten years once you have had a primary vaccination. Review your status with your doctor each year. If you step on a sharp object and it goes through your skin, or if your skin is punctured outdoors, you may need a tetanus booster shot. Always notify your doctor of any such injuries and ask if you need a booster.

If you need to have vaccinations for travel to a specific area, get them at least one month before you depart. That way, you'll have time to deal with any effects they have on your blood sugar control. Your travel agent and health professional can help you research what shots you might need.

Seeing the solutions in front of you in black and white takes much of the stress out of challenges. Attitude is everything!

chapter ten

stress: the tiger you don't want in your tank

Many years ago I read that there are only two choices: love or fear. Back then that idea seemed a bit simplistic, but time and life have changed my mind.

There's the story of a young man who completed a heroic journey and found himself standing in front of two doors. One door concealed a beautiful maiden, the other, a ferocious tiger. The hero knew he had to choose one of the doors, but he had no way of knowing which door would bring forth the maiden and which would release the tiger. For me, the two doors the young hero faced represent fear and love.

When a difficult situation arises, whether it's being late for an important meeting, or something as consistently challenging as living with a chronic illness, many of us choose the door marked "Fear." The fear may be, "I'll make my boss mad," "I'll lose the account," or "I'll never be able to handle all these diet restrictions and new information." Fear rises when we find ourselves in a circumstance for which we feel unprepared. Up against a wall. No way out. Pushed, cornered, helpless. The moment the thoughts and feelings of fear take over, we have chosen the tiger—the tiger called stress. This tiger is ferocious indeed; it has the ability to do great harm to our bodies and our lives. You may think you can't avoid stress, but you actually can learn to choose the other door. You just need to have the right keys (tools) and practice using them.

what's behind the two doors?

To understand what happens when you feel stressed, it helps to know a little about the autonomic nervous system. It controls all of your body's normally involuntary processes, including respiration, heart rate, blood pressure, metabolism, and body temperature. Its two main branches are the sympathetic and the parasympathetic.

When you feel stressed, the brain activates the sympathetic nervous system to speed up your bodily functions, preparing you for action with the fight-or-flight response. The body releases adrenaline. The blood vessels contract, the heart beats faster, blood pressure goes up, and the liver releases sugar and fat into the bloodstream. Adrenaline makes the blood platelets stickier, so the blood will clot more quickly if we're wounded. You're in survival mode and the body is ready for action.

The fight-or-flight response is essential if you need to run away from a lion in the jungle, but it's a tremendous drain on your inner resources if you're in that state much of the time. In our fast-paced culture, many of us are activating the fight-or-flight response almost continuously. The resulting higher blood pressure, extra sugars and fats in the blood, and stickier platelets make us prime candidates for heart disease, stroke, and diabetes. During stress the adrenal cortex releases the steroid cortisol. Cortisol influences weight gain, affects sleep patterns, and suppresses the immune system, making you more susceptible to diseases like cancer. Excessive cortisol can destroy brain cells in the hippocampus, the part of the brain associated with memory and learning.

By comparison, the parasympathetic nervous system calms us down. It's also known as the rest-and-digest response. When it's activated, we feel good. The heart rate drops, blood pressure falls, and respiration slows and deepens. We feel it when we slow down, have a good laugh, go on vacation, or sleep well.

Living with diabetes is a complex challenge. It requires that we learn new physical habits and disciplines. When you add the psychological and emotional issues of chronic illness, it's easy to feel stressed. Even though the fight-or-flight response is built into us, we can learn to calm it down. In every moment, we do have a choice. Actually, we have two choices.

choices

When a scientific theory offers a compact explanation for a wide range of phenomena, it is described as being *elegant.* Derived from the Latin *elegare,* *e* meaning "out" and *legare* meaning "to choose or select," the word "elegant" means to choose or select out of many possibilities. It implies simplicity and gracefulness. To deal with the stress of diabetes, I offer you the simplicity of, "You have two choices."

Diabetes represents a loss of control. Most people with diabetes can't choose whether we have it or not, but there are still many choices to be made. My son, Brennan, loved food and when he was first diagnosed, I was worried that the restricted diet would cause problems. The dietitian told me, "Just be sure to give him choices at each meal and snack. Don't put only your choice in front of him. Let him retain a small measure of control."

Concerning diabetes, you have two choices. You can take care of your diabetes—or not. Of course, most people take care of their diabetes, but perhaps not as consistently as they could. Yet merely becoming aware of the fact that they're making a choice can be a step in the right direction. Each day, each meal, we have the chance to observe which choice we've made. It's a simple "either/or"; either we did what we know is best or we didn't. We don't have to berate ourselves or pass judgments on the choices we've made. Becoming conscious of a choice can often lead to making better choices at another time.

I made a New Year's resolution to "seek what was beneficial." Each time I considered an activity or a meal or a conversation, I asked myself "Is this beneficial?" I lost track of the question after several weeks and am starting to use it again, with good results. I find that merely asking the question keeps me aware of my goals regarding food, exercise, and my state of mind.

Your question might be "Is this helping me control my diabetes?" You might notice that you could be making better choices, but something seems to be getting in your way. What then?

You have two choices. You can look more closely at why you're not doing what you know you should . . . or not! Looking more closely can help you choose differently. You can't change what you can't see. If you look more closely at the "why" of your choice, you have two choices of where to look: the mind or the body.

the merry-go-round mind

The mind produces thoughts and images. Most of the time it's on automatic pilot, connecting the dots of our days, rehashing yesterday's news. It's estimated that more than 95 percent of the thoughts we think are recycled. It's a merry-go-round of mental activity with rarely a brass ring in sight. New experiences are most often filtered through perceptions we've accepted as true. Yet, most of these perceptions haven't been examined to see if they're appropriate or beneficial.

A young woman had just returned from her honeymoon and was preparing a meal for her husband. He walked into the kitchen as she was cutting off the end of the ham before she put it in the roasting pan. He asked her why she was doing that.

She said, "Because that's what you do."

"No, I don't think so," he responded.

"Well, that's what my mom always does," she answered.

"That doesn't make sense. Call your mom and ask her why she does that."

The young bride called and her mother said, "I do that because that's what you do. That's what your grandma always did."

The husband asked his wife to call her grandmother and ask why she cut off the end of the ham. Her grandmother replied, "Oh, I had this small roasting pan and that was the only way I could fit it in."

Suppose you are unsure of yourself in a certain area, because you were picked on by family or friends as a child, and lost confidence in your abilities. Someone says something constructive to be helpful and because of your insecurity, you choose to focus on the suggestion as a criticism, a message that what you're doing is not good enough. Yet the same constructive suggestion made to a person who has confidence in that area would probably elicit a "Thank you, that's a good idea." Same suggestion, two different experiences. As William Shakespeare said, "There's not a thing, but thinking makes it so."

To apply that concept to living with diabetes, we can paraphrase baseball legend Yogi Berra, "Diabetes is like baseball; it's 95 percent mental and the other half is physical." Using that formula, 95 percent of what you think about diabetes is half your battle. With regard to your thoughts about having diabetes and managing it, guess what? You have two choices.

You can think positive thoughts or negative thoughts. Negative thoughts will make diabetes seem more difficult. I can't imagine that you'd want diabetes to be any more difficult than it already is, so I'll focus on how to move away from them.

to be or not to be

To deal with the difficulty of negative thoughts, you have two choices. You can let them lead you around like a goat on a rope, or you can consciously replace them with more positive images.

Suppose you hear yourself saying, "I can't stay on a diet all the time. This is impossible!" In that moment, remind yourself of what Henry Ford said, "Whether you think you can or you think you can't—you are right." So you have a choice. You can rephrase the negative thought with an acknowledgement of the truth, "I'm having difficulty staying on my meal plan for every meal." Or an even more positive, "I stay on my meal plan 75 percent of the time and it's possible I can do better."

What a difference changing our thoughts can make! Consider Murphy's Law, "If anything can go wrong, it will." Now imagine replacing it with Maxwell's Law," Nothing is as hard as it looks; everything is more rewarding than you expect; and if anything can go right, it will and at the best possible moment." We see what we look for. Imagine repeating Maxwell's Law to yourself every morning. How much brighter each day would be if you actively looked for and noticed the good in every event and person. Even in diabetes. (Okay, nobody does that all the time, but the more you do it, the happier you'll be. Abraham Lincoln observed, "Most men are about as happy as they make up their minds to be." He knew the territory well. He spent much of his adult life plagued by depression.)

When it comes to negative thoughts, you can become aware of what you're thinking and saying about the challenge of diabetes, and then make an effort to shift the negative to a positive. You even have two choices when it comes to positive thoughts. You can think them and let them go, or you can resolve to use them as inspiration for change. Abe Lincoln also said, "Always bear in mind that your own resolution to succeed is more important than any other one thing."

Shifting a thought, even a positive one, to a resolution is the beginning of change. So the negative, "I can't . . ." can shift to the neutral, "I haven't been . . ." then to the resolution, "I will make the effort to . . ."

acting as if

Another choice for softening stress is to pay attention to the body's response. The body expresses itself through action and feelings. It is possible to change your mood by changing your actions. You can do it by "acting as if." As an actress on a daytime drama, I had a lot of experience "acting as if." As a friend of mine says, "Just because everything seems to be going down the old Tidy-Bowl doesn't mean I have to go there too."

Say you're feeling moody, negative, and miserable. You can act as if you're not. You might put on a comedy show and enjoy a good laugh, or go out with good friends for dinner and a movie. It's the "whistle a happy tune" method. We do it when we have to. It might be you're feeling stressed, but tonight is your son's birthday party and you make a decision that you're going to have a good time, darn it!

Research has shown that when we pretend we're having a good time, we often do. Sometimes the simplest things make a difference. One study found that when people held a pencil between their teeth so that it protruded out of the corners of their mouth, their lips curved up slightly into a smile. As they held the pencil in place, they began to feel better. Smiling tightens the facial muscles (instant face-lift!) and constricts the flow of blood to the sinus area and thus to the brain. A cooler flow of blood is associated with pleasant feelings. You can "Put on a Happy Face" (or stick a pencil in your mouth) the next time difficult feelings arise and see what happens. Exercise is also a terrific mood lightener; so if you feel droopy, try going on a long walk.

Feelings and thoughts work together like partners in a marriage—for better or worse. We sometimes let them drag us into activities we know are not beneficial. Say you're in the habit of having three cups of coffee with sugar at breakfast or a dessert after every dinner. Now that you have diabetes, these patterns of behavior are not a good idea anymore. Regarding an unfortunate habit: You have two choices. You can let it continue, or you can change it.

Of course, the thought of changing a habit may leave you feeling deprived. A habit is a rut in your life's road that has worn down into a comfortable pattern. Habits actually create neurological pathways in the brain. Each time we travel that same path, we reinforce it. If you want to, you can decide that you're the one running the show and you're no longer going to be controlled by an addiction (which is what some habits become).

One way to change a habit is to "forget" it. "For" means "in place of" and "get" means "to procure." To forget a habit requires putting something else in its place. I watched my husband do that recently. He knew he was drinking too much coffee in the morning. He found an herbal tea that he loved, and now he starts each morning with his special tea and doesn't even miss the coffee. By using substitution, you can avoid the feeling of deprivation and also avoid strengthening the old pathways in the brain. It's the same as replacing a negative thought with a positive one. You don't deprive yourself of thinking; you merely improve the outcome of the process.

In paying close attention to your habits and all the changes that may need to be made, you might find it tempting to have a "Pity Party." The mind can be really creative when it comes to feeling sorry for itself. If you find yourself getting caught up in guilt, regret, or judgment, here's a slight rewrite of the words of legendary basketball coach John Wooden, "Do not let what you cannot do, *and do not do,* interfere with what you can do." (The italicized words are mine.)

working with breath, body, and mind

"Life is difficult." These words begin M. Scott Peck's classic book, *The Road Less Traveled.* He's right. It doesn't matter what social status, financial situation, or good intentions you have. Difficulties will come your way. Losses will accumulate. At the end of this life, you and I will have to leave everything behind. So I figure the sooner I stop whining, the better.

I remember many years ago when I decided I didn't want to suffer so much anymore. From the outside my life probably looked great, but on the inside I was a mess. I knew it was time for a change. One of the beneficial things I did for myself was to begin taking yoga classes and studying yoga philosophy. That was fifteen years ago. I have calmed some of the inner turmoil and no longer feel like a sparkler waiting for a match. I have tools and understandings that have made my life easier. Difficulties still arise, but I now know how to meet them. The secret lies in bringing the breath, the body, and the mind into alignment. There are many excellent books written about this subject, so I'll offer a short introduction to these concepts.

the breath

We've all heard "Take a deep breath." It is wise advice. The sages who created the ancient system of philosophy known as yoga understood that if you control your breath, you can control your response to life's challenges. Every breath you take has the potential to shift your body's state of tension or relaxation.

The breath affects the autonomic nervous system. The inhalation inspires the sympathetic nervous system, the let's-get-up-and-get-going response.

The exhalation encourages the parasympathetic nervous system, the let's-relax-and-enjoy-ourselves response. When the inhalation and exhalation are deep and equal in length, the body is able to balance energy and alertness with a relaxed ease.

The first secret to releasing stress is to feel as if the whole body is breathing. Have you ever watched a baby breathe while it's sleeping? Its body expands with the inhalation and softly contracts with the exhalation. When we breathe deeply, we use the diaphragm: the dome shaped muscle that lies between the chest cavity and the pelvic cavity. When we choose stress, the stomach tightens. This disrupts the flow of the breath, making it shorter and shallower, and activates the sympathetic nervous system with its fight-or-flight response. Deep, diaphragmatic breathing massages the vagus nerve that travels from the brain through the diaphragm to the lower organs. Due to this gentle massage, deep breathing can trigger a cascade of calming effects.

When you consciously and deliberately take a few deep breaths, you allow the body to slow down and soften. Through the use of simple techniques such as deep, balanced breathing, you can soften your response to many stressful events. Try this:

✦   Take a deep breath in through your nose. Allow the breath to travel down along the spine toward your tailbone. Exhale long through your nose.

✦   With the next breath, count the length of a comfortable inhalation, perhaps four, five, or six counts. Don't force. Just observe.

✦   Exhale to the same count, through your nose.

✦   Again inhale to that count and allow yourself an equal exhalation.

✦   Once more inhale and exhale, equally. Let your breath return to normal.

My sister attended a talk on women's health given by a famous oncologist. Toward the end of his talk, he said that because of the immediate and definitive impact that proper breathing has on the health of the body, he predicted within in five years health professionals will be recommending breathing exercises. I hope so.

the body

The body experiences stress both as a physical state and as feelings and emotions. The word "emotion" means to move out, stir up, and agitate. Emotions are often experienced as sensations in the body. We may feel sadness in the heart space. We say, "My heart is broken." Fear or anxiety often manifests in the stomach area. We describe it as having "butterflies," or we may feel nauseous. When difficult feelings arise, our tendency is often to want to put them aside and ignore them. We march on, good little soldiers. Of course, looking the other way doesn't make them disappear. They're still there, gnawing away at us.

Getting these feelings out in the open in a constructive way makes them much less powerful. It's the "bogeyman in the closet" approach. He's really big and scary until Mom opens the closet door and turns the light on so we can see he's not in there in the first place.

There are many good ways to shine a little light on the subject. You begin by becoming aware that you are experiencing feelings that are not comfortable or peaceful. Bringing awareness to a feeling is the beginning of change. Then bring it more fully into the light. Talk with a friend or health care professional, preferably one who is a good listener and understands something about your situation. Talking about your feelings helps you better define them and see more clearly where they might be coming from.

You might get a few pieces of paper and write nonstop for fifteen to twenty minutes, pouring out whatever is parading around inside. Then read them aloud to yourself. Those feelings and thoughts will often seem more manageable when you hold them in your hand. You can then decide which feelings have valid reasons behind their existence and which ones are based on FEAR—False Evidence Appearing Real. You can shift your feeling state by bringing the breath and body into harmony:

✦ Begin with three deep breaths, inhaling through the nose and exhaling through gently pursed lips.

✦ Take a few moments to bring your awareness to your body and notice how you are feeling. You notice, "I'm feeling anxious."

Continue breathing slowly and deeply and let the mind recount which thoughts or events contributed to the anxious feeling. Become aware of where the anxiety is affecting your body. Perhaps your stomach feels jittery or you feel heaviness around your heart. Just notice it; don't try to change it.

✦ Now imagine inhaling into the center of the feeling and that area of the body, allowing it to be warmed by the breath. Exhale from the center of that area, allowing it to soften. Breathe consciously for a few moments, allowing the body to expand with the warm inhalation and soften with the exhalation.

the mind

The mind can travel to thoughts that are not in your best interest. Writer Anne Lamott wryly observed, "My mind is a neighborhood I do not want to go into alone." Sometimes the mind projects into the future, perhaps imagining a traumatic situation. It's then very easy to be swept along by worry and fear. We forget that what inspired the negative feelings has not even occurred. It's only a projection of our imagination and may, in fact, never occur.

This happened a few years ago to my sister, Peggy. A person in her department made a big mistake and they were in danger of losing a very important account. Peggy was in a tailspin, imagining that her boss might fire her over the loss of the account. As we talked through her fears, she saw that there was only a partial chance the account would be lost and that her boss would fire her because of that. Even if he did, she realized she could find another job, possibly an even better one. Having allayed her fears, she was able to talk calmly with her boss. She explained how the mistake had occurred and how her department could prevent it from occurring again. He was impressed with her assessment and her solution. She wasn't fired. She imagined an outcome that didn't happen.

An article in *Spirituality and Health Magazine* reported on the importance of giving "Verbal First Aid" in emergency situations. It noted that the words spoken by a first responder could help save a life by calming and encouraging a severely injured person. In living with diabetes, the mind is the first responder, the first paramedic on the scene, when things get tough. The mind can be like a puppy we adopted. From the first day we brought him home, he ran from room to room, making messes and creating chaos. I was no match for his energetic destructiveness and after two days, I took him back to the breeder. I later learned about "crate training," sequestering a puppy for periods of time during the day to keep it under surveillance and closely guide its activities. We can learn to "crate train" the mind, taking it from troublesome thoughts and sequestering it in a quiet place to get it under control. That way, we keep it from creating inner chaos.

Crate training for the mind begins by becoming aware of what the mind is creating. Several years ago, I attended a meditation workshop. One of its goals was to develop a greater awareness of our inner state. We had been instructed to practice directing our attention inward, both during the sessions and on our breaks. When we'd come back from a break, the leader would ask us, "What are you looking at?" Each time he asked that, I realized that rather than directing my attention inward, my eyes were skittering around the room while my mind spewed observations and judgments. "She has such a pretty face. He needs a haircut. I need to call my sister and tell her about . . ."

His question gave me a tool to examine where my mind was leading me. I went home determined to put it to use. One morning as I sat for meditation, I found myself struggling with an unresolved problem. I realized what I was doing and chided myself, *Gloria, what are you looking at? It's a beautiful morning. Your bills are paid. Your children are fine. You and your husband are happy together. Stop fussing about that old problem.*

I brought my awareness back to the breath, but immediately my mind began sweeping over its memory like a proofreader looking for mistakes. I watched as it once again settled on that unresolved problem. This was getting annoying. I told myself to put the matter aside, but no sooner had I taken another breath, then my mind flew to its perch and began pecking at the same old issue. If I'd been in a cartoon, at that moment a light bulb would have appeared over my head: "Wow! I have a negative mind!" Here I was in a beautiful, peaceful setting, but my mind wanted to hang around the only sore spot it could find.

What a shock! I had always thought I was a person who looked at the bright side of life. If you had informed me that my mind gravitated toward negativity I would have argued, "No, no, I'm a very positive person." Yet I had just witnessed my mind's tendency to search for trouble. Instead of looking at all that was right with my life that morning, my mind was looking at the one thing it could find that was wrong.

When diabetes is causing you stress or fear, you can ask yourself, "What am I looking at?" How is your mind framing your experience of diabetes in that moment? Is it daydreaming of all the fearful things that could happen?

Here's the truth: *You don't have to believe everything you think.* The mind sometimes creates stories that are not true. Stories that most likely never will be true.

As soon as you become aware that thoughts or ideas are causing upset or stress, just drop them. I recently cut the back of my leg on a jagged piece of plastic while getting out of a kayak, and several days later it looked a little red along the sides of the wound. My thoughts quickly skipped from "It could be infected" to, "What if it got infected and then I got gangrene? I wonder what it would be like to have an artificial leg?"

My drama queen mind saw the cut on my leg and turned me into an amputee! As soon as I heard what I was thinking, I didn't even give myself time to attach any worry to the idea. I shifted from negative to positive. I reminded, *re-minded*, myself that my body knows how to heal itself. (I also did the practical thing and had someone look at the wound to make sure it wasn't infected.)

The next time some aspect of diabetes threatens you with mental stress, try *re-minding* yourself. Use your awareness to notice what you are looking at. Then put the great gift of free will to work and choose to think what gives you peace.

using the intelligence of the heart

Through the centuries, saints and sages have described the heart as the seat of wisdom. In everyday speech, we use the word "heart" to denote more than the physical pump. We think of it as our essence or core. We have a "heart to heart" talk or get "to the heart of the problem." I say I'm "broken-hearted" or I "didn't have the heart for it" or something "touched my heart."

In Chinese medicine, the heart is considered a vital substance or life-energy that houses the connection between body and mind. It's the residence of *Shen* (mind or spirit) and communicates messages throughout the body through the blood vessels. Native Americans believe the heart is a bridge between earth and sky, and that our hearts must stay open to both the practical and the mystical.

The ancient Judaic tradition identifies the heart as one of the *Sefirot*, the energy centers of the body. This center is known as *Tiffer et*—beauty, harmony, and balance. The Kabbalah describes the heart as the central sphere that holds the key to health and well-being. This sounds similar to the teachings of Yoga philosophy, which recognize the heart as the seat of individual consciousness and equilibrium. In the language that Jesus spoke, Aramaic, the word for heart, *leba*, means the center of feeling and intelligence.

Recent research is confirming these ideas. We think of the heart as the center of feeling, but the brain houses all our intelligence, right? No. Researchers have discovered that the heart has its own independent nervous system and is capable of making its own decisions. Physiologists John and Beatrice Lacey of the Fels Research Institute noticed that when the brain sends messages to the heart, the heart does not automatically obey. In fact, the heart sends more messages to the brain than the brain sends to the heart. It has its own language, which the brain obeys. In a very real sense, the heart has a mind of its own! (Good song title.) Research is now confirming what the poets have been saying for centuries: the heart plays an important role in emotional experience.

Other clues indicate that the intelligence of the heart is meant to have primacy. In a developing fetus, the heart begins beating before the brain is even formed. The emotional centers, such as the amygdala and hippocampus, emerge from the brain stem first and then the thinking brain grows around the emotional centers. The heart doesn't even need the brain in order to beat. The source of the heartbeat is within the heart.

If you have any doubts that the heart's intelligence was meant to have precedence, consider this: the magnetic field produced by the heart is five thousand times greater than the field produced by the brain. The heart's field can be measured many feet away from the body and can be detected in the brain waves of other people near us, but the magnetic field produced by the brain can only be measured an inch or so outside the skull.

We think of the heart pump and the metaphorical, emotional heart as different and separate, yet research has shown that the physical and meta-physical heart interact. The ways in which the heart communicates to the brain and the rest of the body has led researchers to postulate that the heart is linked to a higher intelligence.

HeartMath

Doc Childre and The HeartMath Institute have spent many years researching the ways we can access this higher intelligence of the heart and put it to use to help regulate our emotional states and reduce stress. They've developed three basic tools that have been astonishing in their effectiveness.

Dr. Paul J. Rosch, President of the American Institute of Stress and Clinical Professor of Medicine and Psychiatry, New York Medical College commented, "HeartMath is a unique stress reduction system that is unusually effective for reducing anxiety and improving performance. Unlike many other services and products that make similar claims, it has a solid scientific basis, and has been thoroughly tested in a variety of settings that have clearly demonstrated these benefits."

The three tools detailed in the book *The HeartMath Solution* are being used by top health care companies, schools, and international corporations and have produced significant results. For example, employees were taught the HeartMath techniques at one hospital and employee turnover was reduced from 28 percent to 5.9 percent Motorola manufacturing facilities employees increased productivity by 93 percent A Royal Dutch Shell executive had the first normal blood pressure reading in fifteen years.

The impact of a one-day HeartMath workshop on 1,400 people at six global companies was pooled. One day of training achieved these results, which were being sustained after six months:

✦   60 percent reduction in anxiety

◆ 41 percent reduction in intent to leave the job
◆ 24 percent improvement in the ability to focus
◆ 45 percent reduction in exhaustion
◆ 25 percent improvement in listening ability

The HeartMath tools are based on research in the relatively new field of neurocardiology. These tools—*Freeze-Frame*, the *Heart Lock-in*, and *Cut-Thru*—help people tap into their inherent "heart intelligence," moving from the chaotic state that stress creates into a state of physical, mental, and emotional coherence.

The word "coherence" means "the quality of being logically integrated, consistent, and intelligible." We all know this feeling. It's when we're working in a focused, harmonious way. Everything seems to flow. We're on our game. Athletes call it "the zone," when they're functioning at their highest level—mind, body, and heart in sync. Gabriella Boehmer of the HeartMath Institute notes, "Being in 'the zone' does not have to be a random event. You can learn how to create that coherence."

That's where the HeartMath tools step in. They provide ways to move away from stress and its allies—frustration, fear, anxiety, and anger—toward coherence. A report from the World Health Organization and International Diabetes Federation recently underscored the need for "whole person approaches to patient care" and the importance of psychological well-being in people who have diabetes. A recent study of patients with diabetes remarked on evidence that patients' perceptions and stress management styles "may substantially influence clinical status." Coping with stress by becoming angry, anxious, and emotional or through detachment and denial can adversely affect blood sugar control. Furthermore, studies published in the *Canadian Journal of Diabetes Care* and *Diabetes Care* have shown that significant relationships exist between effective self-care and long-term blood sugars (HbA1c).

the tools

Each of the HeartMath tools provides an important aspect of emotional self-management. *Freeze-Frame* is the most basic tool, allowing a person to step back from stressful situations and emotionally draining reactions and choose wiser responses. *Heart Lock-In* enables one to "lock-in" positive feelings, and to boost energy, efficiency, and peacefulness. *Cut-Thru* addresses recurring emotional patterns, helping to shift away from reactions that are outdated and inappropriate.

Let's take a closer look at *Freeze-Frame*. A motion picture film is made up of thousands of individual frames. In the film industry, "freeze frame" means to stop a film on a single frame to take a closer look. The *Freeze-Frame* technique allows us to call a time-out to take a closer look at what is causing stress. It helps access the heart's intelligence, the intuitive wisdom we possess, so that we can respond in a manner that best serves us—physically, emotionally, and psychologically.

Let me give you an idea of how I used it recently. I received an upsetting email message from an acquaintance. My first impulse was to answer her and correct her thinking. I began feeling anxious about how to clarify my position, conscious of all the fuss it would cause. I remembered a similar conversation with her that had become filled with defenses and rebuttals. Did I really want to engage in another verbal ping-pong match?

I stopped for a moment and used the *Freeze-Frame* technique. I focused my awareness on the area of my heart and took a few quiet breaths. I brought to mind a particularly vivid memory of feeling peaceful—floating in a few inches of the warm ocean water on a sunny day in Hawaii. From this feeling of ease and peace, I asked my heart, "What do I need to know about this that will minimize future stress?"

The answer came instantly. "Stay away."

Well, of course, that was the best thing to do. I let my email upset slip by and saved myself time and energy.

I've been using *Freeze-Frame* for many months now and it's helped me deal with many situations that could have been stressful. The more I've practiced, the easier it has become to access the wisdom of my heart. The five steps of *Freeze-Frame* have been developed over a period of time and are worded very specifically for maximum effect. Although I alluded to the steps in my example above, I won't repeat the exact wording here. If you're interested, it's best that you get the book *The HeartMath Solution* and read, in fullness, the methods, scientific documentation, and success stories.

I had a chance to talk with the Institute's primary researcher, Rollin McCraty, Ph.D. Three years ago, he conducted a pilot study designed to show that the HeartMath tools can be used effectively by people with diabetes to improve their quality of life. He told me, "We knew from extensive experience that these tools work for people, no matter what difficulties they may be having. Yet we felt that they would be especially helpful to those with diabetes, because the lifestyle changes that diabetes demands can be very stressful."

Stress is caused by how we feel about things in our lives. It emanates from our individual perception of those events. An event or circumstance that will be stressful to one person may feel to another like a challenge to be met calmly—yet it's the very same event. How we choose to feel about something (yes, there is an element of choice involved) affects our health.

The introduction at The Institute of HeartMath's website (www.heart math.org) tells us ". . . negative emotions lead to increased disorder in the heart's rhythms and in the autonomic nervous system, thereby adversely affecting the rest of the body. In contrast, positive emotions create increased harmony and coherence in the heart rhythms and improve balance in the nervous system. The health implications are easy to understand: disharmony in the nervous system leads to inefficiency and increased stress on the heart and other organs while harmonious rhythms are more efficient and less stressful . . ."

Dr. McCraty adds, "Emotional stress causes a disorder in the nervous system that taxes systems at the biochemical level of controlling blood sugar. In a generalized way, the sympathetic side of the autonomic nervous system controls the hormonal systems and the parasympathetic controls our immune system. So if we have disharmony in the nervous system, it affects both the hormonal and immune systems."

Freeze-Frame and the other HeartMath tools offer methods to shift our perception of events so that we can move away from reactive, negative patterns of thinking that cause us to feel stressed. In the study Dr. McCraty conducted, the participants found that using the HeartMath tools didn't change their daily hassles of managing diabetes, but the stress they experienced decreased significantly. When the study was over, the staff at the Institute of HeartMath gave a party to thank everyone. Many of the participants brought family members who wanted to find out what had happened to their spouses that changed them so dramatically for the better.

The study also found that there was a significant relationship between practicing the *Heart Lock-In* technique and reduced Hemoglobin A1c (HbA1c) levels. Those who practiced *Heart Lock-In* more frequently lowered their HbA1c levels, whereas those who practiced minimally or not at all had increases in their HbA1c.

one man's experience

Dan Bishop volunteers at the Institute of HeartMath. Dan spent twenty years working his way up to senior vice-president of Packard Bell Electronics. After four and a half years of building it from a one-hundred-thousand-dollar to a billion dollar company, he woke up one morning unable to breathe. It was a wake-up call. Six months later, he left and started his own consulting business, looking for something more fulfilling. He began putting together rejuvenating retreats for executives, and then decided to create an international summit on self-esteem and integrity, gathering experts from around the world. In the process, he met Rollin McCraty who introduced him to the scientific aspects of HeartMath.

Dan told me, "I worked with the Institute for six years, taking their work out into the corporate field. Then three years ago I was diagnosed with MS. *Freeze-Frame* helped me shift my perceptions, control stress, and access deeper parts of myself."

Dan talked at length about how grateful he is to have *Freeze-Frame* and the other HeartMath tools to help him manage the emotional aspects of living with MS. A flare-up of MS is called an exacerbation, which can last for two to three weeks. MS has constant symptoms such as fatigue, but during an exacerbation, a person might find that his arms or legs can't move and his speech becomes slurred.

Like diabetes, the unpredictability of MS can be very stressful. With any exacerbation, there's the possibility of permanent damage, blindness perhaps, or you might wind up in a wheelchair for good. When Dan feels an exacerbation coming on, he uses *Freeze-Frame* to keep himself calm.

He says, "The biggest gift is being able to manage my projections about the future, about my potential demise. I've talked to people with MS about how scary it is, and most don't have the tools to take care of all those thoughts that cause them to worry. You can't give in to hopelessness and depression, because then it's more difficult to take care of yourself and also to ask for help. *Freeze-Frame* helps neutralize the worries and projections. When I use it, my heart reminds me that I am valuable, even though my body isn't functioning as I would like."

Daily limitations, worry, unpredictability, fear about the future—having MS sounds a lot like having diabetes, doesn't it? To learn more about the HeartMath tools and to order *The HeartMath Solution* and other materials, go to www.heartmath.com.

the yoga of relaxation

As a yoga instructor, I have noticed that everyone's favorite part of my classes is the last few minutes, when we practice *savasana*, the corpse pose. The word *yoga* is an ancient Sanskrit word meaning, "yoke together" or "unite." In the posture below, we unite breath, body, and mind in relaxed awareness.

You can read the instructions as you follow them, read them into a tape recorder, and purchase my relaxation CD, *Body, Breath, & Mind*, listed in the Resources for Readers section.

✦ Begin by lying flat on the floor, extending your legs straight down out of your hips and then let your feet flop open to the sides. Let your arms be at the sides of your body with the palms up. Let your head be in alignment with your spine and tuck your chin gently toward your chest to lengthen the back of your neck.

(If your chin and forehead are not level and your chin is jutting up toward the ceiling, place a folded towel under your head. If lying flat on the floor pulls on your lower back, put a thick pillow under your knees so they're bent. This will help release the lower back, so it can relax.)

✦ Gently close your mouth and bring your awareness to your breath. Breathing through your nose, feel the inhalation coming into the nostrils, cool and fresh. Feel the exhalation, warm and soft. Stay with the breath, being fully aware of three consecutive inhalations and exhalations.

✦ Now become aware of your toes, your ankles, and your feet. Let them soften and release—letting go, letting go. Feel the next inhalation and exhalation.

✦ Become aware of your shins and calves, your thighs. Let them soften and release—letting go, letting go. Feel the next inhalation and exhalation.

✦ Become aware of your pelvis, your inner organs, and your buttocks. Let them soften and release—letting go, letting go. Feel the next inhalation and exhalation.

✦ Become aware of your chest, the space around your heart, your shoulders. Let them soften and release, your shoulders settling down away from your ears—letting go, letting go. Feel the next inhalation and exhalation.

✦ Become aware of your fingers, your hands, and arms. Let them soften and release—letting go, letting go. Feel the next inhalation and exhalation.

✦ Now become aware of your face. Unhinge your jaw at the back of your mouth and let there be space between your molars. Let your tongue lie softly in the bottom of your mouth. Find the little muscles at the back of your eyes and let them soften and release. Let your eyes nestle gently into your head—letting go. Let your whole face be as soft as a child's.

✦ Become aware of the brain and let your brain gently soften down away from the inside of your skull, as if it's settling down for a nap.

✦ Bring your awareness to the breath, following the inhalation to its depth and the exhalation to its full length. Rest here, in the breath. If the mind gets busy, gently guide it back to the breath. (Don't judge how many times that happens. Just let go of whatever thought comes as soon as you can and return your awareness to the breath.)

✦ Rest for several minutes. Then bring your knees to your chest and give them a hug, gently stretching your lower back. Roll to your right side and take three deep inhalations and exhalations through your nose. Turn and look down at the floor, bringing your left palm to the floor near your face, and push your body up slowly, followed by your head. Stand up slowly, paying attention to the breath.

If you're at the office or traveling on a plane, you can also follow these basic instructions while seated in a chair.

For a one-minute, mini-*savasana*, breathe through your nose and imagine that you're bringing the breath into the chest and allowing it to encircle the heart. Your inhalation caresses the heart as it comes in and the exhalation releases and softens as it exits. Let your shoulders settle down away from your ears. Let three to five breaths encircle the heart and then return to whatever you were doing.

dr. tim's approach

When Dr. Tim was ten years old, he listened to Earl Nightingale on the radio. Earl presented ideas for focusing our energies to create what we wanted to do or be in our lives. His program was offered on cassette tapes and Dr. Tim wore out two sets of the tapes. Earl's main process involved writing down a problem such as, "My life's a mess. I have Type 2 diabetes and my HbA1c is way too high."

Dr. Tim says, "Then every day you write down twenty ways to improve your life and decrease your HbA1c. It doesn't have to be a different twenty ways each day. If you do this every day for a month, you'll probably have at least a half dozen good ideas that can completely change things."

Dr. Tim uses this technique in his own daily ritual. He writes lists like "twenty ways I can improve my relationship with Kathy" or "twenty ways that I can create memories for our children." One idea he had was to rent a tank of helium at Christmas and allow his children to be creative (with supervision.) They found out that ten fifty-gallon black garbage bags tied together on a rope had almost as much lift as a small hot air balloon and allowed a running child to jump about twenty feet. It was a very memorable day for the whole family, one they still talk about.

Dr. Tim says, "Every major project I have undertaken has involved using this system. Once ideas become focused by writing them down, you often have useful techniques for dealing with the problems that don't seem to have solutions. Seeing the solutions in front of you in black and white takes much of the stress out of challenges. Attitude is everything!"

Diabetes is your own personal IRS, Internal Reality Signal. If you don't pay attention to it now, it will get your attention later, but with fines and penalties added.

chapter eleven

dangers and dragons

My goal in writing this book is to inspire you to be your own best caregiver. Dr. Tim does the same with his patients. You have heard stories of people who've lived successfully with diabetes for thirty, forty, and fifty years. For me, no story feels complete without the hero overcoming insurmountable dangers and invincible dragons. To go the distance with diabetes, it is best that you understand its dangers and know how to outwit them. This chapter details the damage diabetes can do and offers strategies you can use to avoid becoming another statistic. Please don't skip over this chapter. I don't want you to be like some people I have met who've said, "No one told me diabetes could do this to me." People like Danny.

In the winter of 1974 when he was ten, Danny was diagnosed with diabetes. Until he was fifteen or sixteen, he did a good job of taking care of himself. Then he became rebellious, sneaking candy and drinking regular soda. His sister Ann recalls, "I thought of diabetes as manageable. I remember thinking that as long as he seemed to be taking care of himself, everything will be fine."

But things were not fine. At twenty-four, only fourteen years after being diagnosed, Dan began to experience complications. He had hemorrhages in his eyes and had to quit his job as a carpenter's apprentice. Two years later, Dan's doctor put him in the hospital because his kidneys were failing.

He began dialysis, but he had a difficult time. He lost his hair and felt hungry all the time. Then one night, he was coughing violently. Ann told Dan to go to the ER, but he didn't want to go.

Ann says, "I told him 'You need to go to the emergency room and if I'm wrong, too bad.' My dad and I got him to the ER and the doctor told us he was having congestive heart failure. They put him in intensive care."

Dan needed a kidney transplant. Two family members were the best match, Ann and her mother. Ann decided that she would be the one. The night before the surgery, Dan tried to back out, saying he couldn't put his sister through it. For Ann that wasn't an option. In August 1991, Ann gave one of her kidneys to her brother.

After the transplant, other than a minor bout with rejection, Dan thrived. His hair grew back. He bought a motorcycle, much to his mother's dismay. After being sick for so long, he was feeling good, working, having fun. He was developing a serious relationship with a wonderful woman. He bought a house close to his parents, so he could help them when they needed it. Then one evening, while brushing his teeth, Dan had a massive coronary. The paramedics could not revive him. He was twenty-nine years old.

what happened to dan?

When a person with a healthy metabolism eats, the pancreas responds with just the right amount of insulin to keep the blood sugar levels between 80 and 120. When a person with diabetes eats, there is not enough insulin to do the job. Even with diabetes pills or injected insulin, there will be times when the blood sugar is higher than normal.

There was a time when many experts didn't believe that blood sugar levels had anything to do with complications. Then a ten-year study, the Diabetes Control and Complications Trial (the DCCT), was conducted to determine the effect of "tight" blood sugar control. "Tight" control means closely mimicking the body's natural insulin response. Each time food is ingested, the body responds with the exact amount of insulin needed to handle that food. In addition, the body maintains a small constant supply of insulin so that glucose can enter the cells all day and night. For a person with Type 1 diabetes, tight control means taking a shot of short-acting insulin at each meal (or through an insulin pump) and using a long-acting insulin to cover the body's needs over a twenty-four-hour period. The beneficial results of using tight control were so conclusive that the study was discontinued before its ten-year course was completed.

The study demonstrated that those who kept their HbA1c tests below "7" had significantly fewer complications; in some cases, 76 percent fewer complications. Studies of people with Type 2 diabetes in the United States, Japan, and England have also demonstrated that life-threatening complications of diabetes can be significantly reduced (up to 70 percent) when blood sugars are controlled.

Why are normal blood sugars so important?

Diabetes affects practically every tissue in the body. Its complications are largely due to damage to the blood vessels and the nervous system. The effects of higher than normal blood sugar contribute to heart disease and stroke, kidney failure, blindness, nerve damage to organs, and amputation of feet and legs.

Higher than normal blood sugar damages the circulatory system that delivers blood to your organs and cells. It can change cells by a process known as "glycosylation," which means "addition of sugar." Excess glucose and other sugars become chemically attached to molecules in the body. They then undergo chemical changes, forming "advanced glycosylation end-products," or AGEs. These AGEs are dangerous chemical additions to your blood vessels that literally "gum up the works." The longer a person has diabetes with higher than normal blood sugars, the more these mechanisms contribute to the buildup of what researcher Dr. Michael Brownlee calls "biological superglue."

Some of the most serious problems of diabetes are caused by AGEs in blood vessel walls. AGEs are very sticky, so when proteins pass through an area containing AGEs, they can get trapped. As more and more proteins get stuck, the vessel narrows and can't deliver oxygen as it should. When this happens in your leg, it can cause pain while walking, or if it happens in the blood vessels of the heart, it can cause a heart attack. Because AGEs narrow the blood vessels, they seem to play a major role in diabetic kidney disease, eye disease, and heart disease.

Any nerve in your body can be affected by the damage of high blood sugar. Nerve damage is a major factor for impotence in men as well as women, digestive disorders, bowel and bladder problems, loss of feeling in hands and feet, and amputation of limbs.

Research has provided clues as to how high blood sugar causes nerve damage. One way is through biochemical pathways inside and outside your cells that are altered when blood sugar levels increase. An example is a system called the polyol pathway. Glucose in your blood is converted to sorbitol. Your cells do need a certain amount of sorbitol, but too much glucose increases the level of sorbitol and appears to decrease levels of myoinositol, another essential chemical. Scientists have witnessed that nerve damage in diabetic animals is associated with elevated sorbitol and reduced myoinositol levels.

Dr. Michael Brownlee and his team of researchers at Albert Einstein College of Medicine recently identified an enzyme, PARP (poly-ADP-ribose-polymerase) that is activated by high blood sugar. PARP damages blood vessels and contributes to nerve, eye, and kidney damage. His team is working on finding drugs that inhibit PARP.

These complications happen because of higher than normal blood sugar levels. There is no guarantee that you can completely avoid complications. You may take good care of yourself over the years and still have some damage, but if you can choose to conscientiously control your blood sugar levels, you can significantly decrease your risk of complications.

your heart and blood vessels

Darren is a fifty-two-year-old lumber broker who has a history of high blood pressure. He's also smoked a pack a day for thirty years. Dr. Tim often had discussions with Darren about quitting smoking, but Darren said he enjoyed it and "that's that." One night Darren called Dr. Tim complaining of crushing chest pain. He was having a heart attack. He was rushed to the emergency room and stabilized.

Dr. Tim notes, "Darren responded well to angioplasty and stent placement. We also did blood work on him and found he had elevated blood sugar levels. Following these procedures, he quit smoking, which, as his doctor, made me want to jump up and cheer. I started him on oral diabetes medication and his blood glucose was controlled in about a week and a half."

Darren had been living with higher than normal blood sugar and blood pressure levels, plus he smoked. Smoking cigarettes narrows or constricts blood vessels. Smoking and diabetes are a very dangerous combination. Darren understands that now.

Your cardiovascular system pumps blood and delivers oxygen and nourishment to your entire body. It also removes waste products. Problems occur when the walls of the blood vessels thicken, become blocked, and result in poor circulation. Diabetes greatly increases the risk of heart attack or stroke. According to Dr. Barton Stobel at the University of Vermont, people with diabetes have twice the risk of having a heart attack, twice the amount of heart muscle damage from a heart attack, and twice the risk of developing congestive heart failure or dying.

If you have the following conditions, as well as diabetes, you have a significant risk of heart disease:

◆ High blood pressure
◆ Lipid disorders including: high LDL cholesterol, high triglycerides, and low HDL cholesterol
◆ obesity
◆ lack of physical activity

atherosclerosis and peripheral arterial disease

The common ingredient in all heart and blood vessel diseases is a partial or total blockage caused by atherosclerosis, the buildup of plaque deposits. Research has provided clear evidence that both high blood sugar and high blood fat levels are involved in the buildup of plaque. When a blockage prevents blood from reaching the heart, a heart attack results. When it's a blockage of blood to the brain, stroke results. Partial blockage to the large coronary arteries causes chest pain (angina) as sections of the heart are damaged from lack of nutrients.

When fatty deposits of cholesterol clog the arteries leading to the feet or legs, peripheral arterial disease results. Walking, standing, or exercising may become painful. There may also be changes in your skin color or temperature; loss of hair on your toes or feet; change in thickness and appearance of your toenails; abnormal sensations in your feet, legs, thighs, or calves, such as tingling, pins and needles, foot going to sleep, or cramps; and pain in your legs when you walk.

metabolic syndrome

There's also a condition known as "metabolic syndrome," which is closely related to Type 2 diabetes. Twenty-five percent of Americans have this problem and it's increasing. With metabolic syndrome, your body makes insulin, but the cells do not allow all of the insulin to enter, so there are high levels of insulin in the blood vessels. High insulin levels cause vascular inflammation, fat production, and an increase in triglycerides, blood pressure, and waist size. This combination leads to higher risk of heart attacks.

You have the metabolic syndrome if you meet three of the following criteria: blood pressure greater than 130/85; triglycerides greater than 150; fasting glucose levels above 110, and LDL cholesterol below 40 in men and below 50 in women. Waist size is also an indicator if it's greater than 40 inches in men and 35 inches in women. Both metabolic syndrome and Type 2 diabetes are most often the result of your weight, food intake, and exercise routine (or lack thereof.)

Dr. Tim notes, "Metabolic syndrome typically shows itself as high triglycerides and low HDL cholesterol. Also, I've noticed that most of my patients with this syndrome feel chronically tired and constantly hungry. That's because the cells are not getting any nourishment even though insulin is present. A person may not have all these symptoms, but if they have some of them, they should have their blood checked and talk to their physician about metabolic syndrome."

feeling the warning signs

For those with Type 2, there's a strong possibility that diabetes has been undetected for several years, which means it may have already done some damage by the time it's diagnosed. If this is your circumstance, you may not be able to feel the chest pains that are an early warning sign of a heart attack. Yet it's vital that you respond to these early warning signs by going to the hospital immediately. The longer you wait, the more damage the heart attack can do.

The reasons for lack of sensitivity are unknown but may be due to neuropathy. When you are first diagnosed, you will want to discuss your risk factors for heart disease with your caregiver. Do everything in your power to prevent, detect, and treat any problems. Know the warning signs for heart attack and if you think there's a possibility you may be having one, don't delay. Get yourself to the ER immediately.

what you can do

As a person who has diabetes, what can you do to avoid a heart attack or stroke? My mother had both and, believe me, being as disabled as she was is not worth the choices that led to it. You can greatly influence the health of your heart and blood vessels by keeping your diabetes, your blood pressure, and your cholesterol levels in good control. You can choose what is beneficial for your body through what you eat, how much you exercise, how you handle life's challenges (stress), and by choosing not to smoke. If including all these beneficial choices doesn't do the whole job, there are drugs called statins that can add extra assistance.

A study of 2,838 people in Britain and Ireland found that a daily dose of cholesterol-lowering statin dramatically reduced the risk of serious heart disease (by 36%) and stroke (48%) in people with Type 2 diabetes, even those who already had normal cholesterol levels. Statins do not take the place of properly caring for your body, but they are generally safe and effective as an additional means of reducing risk. In fact, just recently researchers have begun recommending that all people with diabetes take a statin as a preventative. This even includes those who have normal LDL cholesterol levels. The one side effect that Dr. Tim has noticed is that sometimes there can be muscle aches and pains. It usually occurs within the first month of taking the statin and the pain goes away once the statin is stopped.

your eyes

In 1985, Bill went to his doctor and discovered he had an elevated blood sugar. As Bill tells it, "The doctor told me I had Type 2 diabetes and had to go on a special diet. I tried to follow the diet, but like most people with diabetes, I did not follow it because it was too hard to do so."

He took oral medications, but they were not working well for him. His physician put him on insulin and he gained back weight he'd lost, but he began to lose his vision. Bill had laser surgery, but the treatments came too late. He said, "The treatments did not help me, because laser surgery only keeps you from going totally blind and does not improve the eyesight."

Bill missed many opportunities to save his sight. He didn't manage his food plan, he didn't test his blood sugar, and he didn't have a yearly eye exam with an expert.

Your eyes are especially vulnerable to the effects of diabetes. High blood sugar causes blurred vision in the early stages of diabetes, but often the blurring is not permanent and disappears once blood sugar is back to normal levels. People with diabetes are also at greater risk to develop glaucoma and cataracts, especially if their blood sugar is not under good control. Long-term high blood sugar changes red blood cells so that they don't move easily through small blood vessels. The cells stiffen and can rupture weakened blood vessels. One of the first places these ruptures may appear is in the eyes.

The most serious eye problem that diabetes can cause is damage to the retina. The retina is a thin, light-sensitive lining in the back of your eye. "Retinopathy" is the word used to describe the damage done to your eye's small blood vessels. Most people who have diabetes for more than twenty-five years exhibit some changes in their retinas. Yet if the changes are diagnosed early and treated promptly and correctly, complete blindness is rare.

There are two stages to retinopathy: an initial stage called non-proliferative retinopathy and a more serious one, proliferative retinopathy, which I briefly mentioned in chapter seven. Another condition called macular edema can occur with either stage. In the initial stage, high blood sugar damages blood vessels in the eye. Fluid leaks occur and cause the retina to swell. Fluid in the central part of the retina causes blurred vision and can be treated with laser surgery.

With proliferative or advanced retinopathy, abnormal blood vessels grow over the retina. They can rupture and bleed into the clear gel that fills the eye. Light is blocked from reaching the retina and loss of vision or blindness results. The blood vessels can also cause scar tissue, which can result in a detached retina.

I mentioned Bill's story to Dr. Jerry Cavallerano at Joslin Diabetes Institute who told me, "His experience reinforces the importance of an annual eye examination for anyone with diabetes. Appropriate laser surgery can reduce the risk of severe vision loss from proliferative diabetic retinopathy to less than 2 percent over a five-year period. Appropriate laser surgery for diabetic macular edema can reduce the risk of moderate vision loss by 50 percent or more."

He also warned that serious eye disease can be present even if there is no change in vision, and that's why it's so important to have a comprehensive eye examination with an ophthalmologist once a year. Laser surgery is most effective if it's performed prior to any loss of vision. The laser does not "cure" diabetic retinopathy, but it can reduce vision loss.

what you can do

Have a dilated eye exam at least once a year. Also check your blood pressure frequently, because high blood pressure increases your risk of retinopathy. If you are diagnosed with retinopathy, your doctor may recommend fundus photography or fluorescein angiography, along with more frequent eye examinations.

Your first line of defense against eye disease is maintaining normal blood sugar readings, along with normal blood pressure and cholesterol levels.

Add these strategies to an annual eye exam and you will go a long way toward protecting your eyesight.

Research is also doing its part to help protect you. Innovative treatments being developed appear to block the growth factors that cause formation of new blood vessels. Another area of research targets the molecular processes involved in diabetes-related complications and attempts to reverse these changes that happen at the cellular level.

Bill, who is now legally blind, now understands that it didn't have to happen. He cautions others with diabetes to, "Keep very close account of your blood sugar and don't overeat. I also stress getting your eye exams every six months to a year." Thanks, Bill.

your kidneys

There was a monk who spent many years in spiritual practice. He lived each day quietly, chopping wood for his fire and carrying water from a nearby spring. After many years of practice, he attained enlightenment. A young novice wanted to know how the monk's life had changed.

The monk answered, "Before enlightenment, chop wood, carry water. After enlightenment, chop wood, carry water."

Joe Gaspar understands the monk's answer. Joe's before and after experience flank a pancreas and kidney transplant. He was diagnosed with diabetes at age twelve in 1974, at a time when the tools of diabetes care were not as refined as they are now.

Joe says, "I went to the doctor once a month for a glucose test which would determine how much insulin I took for the next month. Now we know that's a really poor way to manage diabetes."

In 1996, Joe was told he had kidney failure. He went on dialysis and was assessed as a pancreas and kidney transplant candidate. Then on March 11, 1998, the transplant coordinator called. Joe remembers, "The coordinator said, 'Joe, I've got the organs for you. Come down to the hospital and if all goes well, you can have the transplant tomorrow.'"

Joe recovered well and now leads a very normal life. He married the lovely woman who was with him through his transplant and they recently had their first child. Joe takes good care of himself, just as he did before the transplant five years ago. (Before and after, chop wood, carry water.) Instead of insulin, he takes a combination of anti-rejection medicines, anti-hypertension medicines, and vitamins. He remains physically active, allowing his body the exercise it needs. He drinks plenty of water and chooses to eat low-salt, low-sugar, and low-fat foods. He eats mostly fresh foods, staying away from preservatives and nitrates. Once in a while he enjoys a glass of wine. He follows the same regimen that any diabetes doctor would recommend.

Joe feels certain that if he'd had access to home blood glucose monitoring, the hemoglobin A1c test and the new insulins, he probably would not have had kidney failure diabetes. Joe says, "I think people who have these tools are very fortunate. Now there's increased monitoring, increased awareness, and the medicines are better."

what happened to joe?

Your kidneys function as blood-cleansing organs. They look like two small baking potatoes. Each contains about one million tiny blood vessels, or filters, called nephrons, that wash your blood and discard waste products into your urine.

Over a period of time, high blood sugar blood damages these filtering units until the filtering network starts to collapse and releases waste products into the blood. Symptoms of kidney failure include swelling of the hands, ankles, face, and other parts of the body; loss of appetite; fatigue; skin irritations; confusion; and difficulty controlling blood sugar levels.

The onset of these symptoms can be gradual, but they do signal the loss of kidney function. If you have the early stages of kidney disease you may not experience any symptoms, so it's important for your doctor to test your urine. One test looks for microalbuminuria, tiny amounts of protein in the urine. Another test is for creatinine, a waste product from muscle activity. Normally, your kidneys remove it from your blood, so a buildup of creatinine is another sign that your kidneys are not functioning normally.

If you do have protein or creatinine in your urine, your doctor will begin treating you with medication to protect your kidneys from further damage. You will be advised to get your blood sugar and blood pressure in good control, and may be put on a low-protein diet. Eating a low-protein diet can ease the burden on your kidneys.

Once the kidneys are damaged, they can continue to deteriorate until you must find other ways to cleanse your blood. One is through dialysis, which involves being hooked up to a machine either several times a day or several times a week. The other possibility is a kidney transplant.

Here is the bad news: diabetes is the most common cause of kidney failure in the United State and the rate of kidney failure has been rising in the over-forty-five age group by twelve-fold.

Here is the good news: about 80 percent of those with diabetes don't develop end stage renal disease and live their lives without the complication of kidney failure. A study published in the *New England Journal of Medicine* found that tight control of blood sugar, blood pressure, and cholesterol were effective in reversing early stages of kidney disease. This study emphasizes the importance of early screening and prompt treatment of these factors.

what you can do

There are several strategies you can use to prevent kidney damage. The first is to keep your hemoglobin A1c levels below "7." A large study in Madison, Wisconsin showed there is a significant relationship between kidney failure and higher hemoglobin A1c levels. Also:

- ✦ Have yearly blood tests for BUN, creatinine, and microalbumin.
- ✦ If you have microalbumin, talk with your doctor about taking ACE inhibitor or an ARB.
- ✦ Control your blood sugar.
- ✦ Control your blood pressure.
- ✦ Seek medical help for bladder and kidney infections promptly.
- ✦ Drink plenty of water: eight 8 oz. glasses of water a day. Drink more if blood sugar is elevated or if you have a bladder or kidney infection.

✦ You can also take cranberry pills. They're available from a health store or nutrition store (not the regular juice, as it contains too much sugar). Cranberry helps prevent bacteria from sticking to the walls of the urinary tract.

erectile dysfunction

Dr. Tim has a foolproof method for getting the attention of male patients who have diabetes. When they ask him, "Do I really need to worry about this diabetes stuff?" Dr. Tim holds up his index finger and slowly lets it droop over halfway. Then he says, "This is what you get when you don't take care of your diabetes." They get the picture.

A survey of men with diabetes asked them to rank its complications in order of their importance. Erectile dysfunction (ED) was ranked third, just behind blindness and kidney failure.

Many years ago, an acquaintance had just been diagnosed with diabetes. His doctor was describing the damage that uncontrolled blood sugars can do. My friend found himself fairly cavalier about the doctor's list until he heard the words *erectile dysfunction*.

He quickly responded, "Diabetes can make me impotent?"

"Yes," his doctor replied.

"Okay, Doc. Tell me what I need to do and I'll do it."

From a man's point of view, virility is a big issue. It can be a major contributor to or detractor from a man's self image. In the general population, the causes are most often physical and psychological. Diabetes makes ED more likely as it damages blood vessels and nerves. In addition, some men (and women) experience depression when diagnosed with diabetes.

Sexual function depends on nerve and blood vessel health. When there is sexual stimulus, nerves signal small valves to fill the penis with blood. They then close and trap the blood, keeping the penis erect. When the stimulus subsides, the blood drains out. ED may be due to damage of the nerve fibers that control these valves. It may also be due to narrowing or thickening of the blood vessels, blocking the blood flow to the penis.

women, too . . .

Poorly controlled diabetes can also affect a woman's sex life. It contributes to vaginal dryness, causing uncomfortable sexual relations. Higher than normal blood sugar makes a woman more susceptible to vaginal yeast infections. Menstruation can cause a rise in blood sugar levels for a few days before the monthly flow. Chronically high blood sugar may also cause a delay in the onset of puberty and create menstruation irregularities.

There was a time when a woman with diabetes was told not to have children. Because of the great tools we now have for achieving tight control, that is no longer the case. The bodily changes of pregnancy make consistent, meticulous care essential, but a woman who has diabetes can have a healthy baby.

If you're thinking about starting a family, find a doctor who specializes in pregnancy in women with diabetes. Work with your doctor to get your blood sugars in a normal or near normal range (an HbA1c below 6.5) for at least 2–3 months before you become pregnant. Also, get a complete check of your eyes and kidneys before you try to become pregnant.

Once you are pregnant, work with your doctor and diabetes educator to adjust your diet and add insulin as needed. Diabetes pills cannot be used to control blood sugar, because they cross the placenta and cause hypoglycemia in the fetus. Many women decide to use an insulin pump during pregnancy. Discuss it with your doctor.

Both men and women with poorly controlled diabetes are also more prone to urinary tract infections. When blood sugar is high, the immune system is less effective in destroying bacteria.

what can you do?

ED usually appears gradually after a number of years of poorly controlled blood sugar. Studies have shown that the degree of blood sugar control has a strong correlation to the early development of ED. Other contributing factors include smoking, obesity, lack of exercise, and alcohol use. These are factors you can influence.

At the first sign of changes in your sexual functioning, talk with your doctor. Sometimes ED can be caused by medications you're taking. If you are a woman experiencing uncomfortable sexual relations, your doctor may prescribe lubricants or medications. For men, the doctor may check your sex hormone levels or suggest an evaluation from a urologist, a urinary tract specialist. You may also be advised to see a psychologist to help you sort through stresses in your life, which can be a contributing factor.

New treatments like Viagra, Levitra, and Cialis have enjoyed widespread acceptance and have shown relatively few side effects. The success rate of these drugs is 35 percent in men with diabetes and 70 percent in the general population. One caution: Men with coronary artery disease who are taking nitrates should not take these drugs. (Remember Jack Nicholson in *Something's Gotta Give?*) These drugs dilate blood vessels and so do nitrates—not a good combination. A rare side effect is sudden blindness that can be permanent.

Please be aware that although taking a drug for ED may solve the symptom, you and your doctor may want to search for the underlying causes of ED.

nerve damage

Nerve damage (neuropathy) can be very painful and debilitating. Researchers aren't exactly sure of how neuropathy develops, but there are some very good clues. Most of the body's cells require insulin to open the cell doors so that sugar can enter to create energy. Nerves are different—they do not require insulin's help. If sugar is high in the blood it will be high within the nerve cells also. A covering called Schwann cells surrounds nerves. High blood sugar can cause them to swell and squeeze the nerves. When nerves are unable to send signals the way they should, many problems can result.

There are two types of nerve damage. *Sensory neuropathy* is the result of damage to nerves that affect sensation. It can cause feet and legs to tingle, feel numb, burn, ache, or throb. Or cuts and injuries may go unnoticed, because no pain signals are being sent. Sensory neuropathy can range from minor discomfort to severe pain. If untreated, the pain will go away—not because the condition is better, but because the nerves are dead. If the nerves are dead, you may not recognize injuries like a blister or cut. Nerves send impulses that help preserve muscle tone. Muscle can also waste away due to nerve damage. You may lose muscle in your thighs or feet, making it difficult to rise from a chair or walk.

Autonomic neuropathy affects the nerves that control your organs. It can interfere with automatic bodily activities like heart rate, digestion, and elimination.

When the nerves controlling your digestive tract are affected, gastroparesis results. It's a condition in which the emptying of the stomach is delayed and food just sits there for hours. This causes a feeling of fullness for hours after a meal is eaten. It also causes bloating, pain, nausea, and vomiting. Food and acid may back up into the esophagus, leading to heartburn. Gastroparesis is a very debilitating complication.

If you experience any of the warning signs above, do two things. First, call your doctor and ask for a referral to a GI (gastrointestinal) specialist right away. Secondly, heed the advice of gastroneurologist Dr. Terence Lewis, "Keep your blood sugars under really tight control, if you possibly can, to avoid any further damage."

what can you do?

One more time: keep your blood sugars under control. Many people say that the pain of neuropathy lessens when their blood sugar level is near the normal range. Good blood sugar control has been shown to decrease neuropathies by 60 percent. Alcohol increases neuropathy symptoms, including pain in the feet. A note: when blood sugar control is improved, nerve regeneration can initially cause tingling and discomfort, but that's a good sign!

Also, inform your doctor of any changes in sensation: tingling, pain, or numbness. If you have damage to the nerves that control contraction of your blood vessels, you may get dizzy when you stand up from a seated or lying position. Let your doctor know. If anything changes with your urinary control, digestion, or elimination, call your doctor. There are new treatments for neuropathy. Anytime you experience changes in your body's functions, let your doctor know.

your feet

Several years ago, I was a guest speaker at a diabetes seminar and met a woman who had lost several toes on her left foot. She said, "I've only had diabetes for seven years and I know this is my fault. I'm a nurse and I knew better, but I just didn't take good enough care of myself. I'm doing that now."

People with diabetes spend more days in the hospital with foot problems than any other complication. There are many reasons for this. Diabetes can cause nerve damage and loss of sensation, and narrowing of blood vessels to the lower limbs. With less sensation, an injury can occur and go unnoticed, resulting in infection. Those with poorly controlled diabetes have a higher risk of infection and heal more slowly. If a person with diabetes is older, has limited eyesight, or is significantly overweight, they may not be able to properly examine their feet. A small cut could become an ulcer, leading to gangrene and loss of that limb.

In most cases, foot infections, ulcers, and amputations can be prevented, reduced, or even eliminated if people receive appropriate education and care guidelines. A 1990 study of eighty amputations showed that sixty-nine of them were preventable if proper foot care procedures had been followed.

First of all, wash your feet in warm soapy water every day. Pick a time, maybe first thing in the morning or just before bed, and make foot care part of your hygiene ritual, like brushing your teeth. Before you put your feet in the water, test it to make certain it is not hot. Rinse and dry your feet carefully, being certain to dry between your toes. Don't soak your feet, as it softens the skin and can make it more susceptible to infection. Massage in moisture restoring cream. Nivea, Alpha Keri, and Eucerin Plus are good choices. Udderly Smooth cream is greaseless and stainless. You can call 1-800-345-7339 for information about buying it in your area or go to www.uddercream.com.

Don't use a perfumed lotion and don't put lotion or cream between your toes. If your feet perspire, use a little talcum, baby powder, or mild foot powder to absorb moisture, but again, don't put it between your toes.

File your toenails. File them just to the end of your toes, not too short. Don't use scissors or clippers as you might cut yourself, leading to infection.

Inspect your feet every day. What are you looking for?

✦ **Color:** Your skin color should look normal. Look for red, white, or blue areas. White means not enough blood is getting to an area. Blue signals a bruise, blood under the skin, or could be the beginning of an ulcer. Red signals an inflammation. Redness anywhere, but especially over bones, is not desirable. Redness on the top of the foot is almost always due to poorly fitted shoes. Redness on the bottom can be due to poor fit or poor circulation. Your feet should always be free of any pressure areas.

✦ **Temperature:** Your feet should feel warm all over. Increased warmth is a sign of infection. A cool or cold area means poor circulation.

✦ **Sensation:** Can you feel a gentle touch on the top and bottom of foot through your socks? Do you have any numbness or tingling?

✦ **Painful areas**

✦ **Sores, cuts, scratches, or breaks in skin**

✦ **Change in hair:** Do you have hair on your lower legs and toes? Where does it stop? Hair loss indicates poor circulation.

✦ **Dry skin**

✦ **Calluses and discoloration under a callus:** If a callus forms, it's a sign of pressure and potential ulcers. Do not cut corns or calluses. Do not use corn- or callus-removal products. Corns and calluses should be examined regularly by your doctor or a podiatrist (foot specialist).

✦ **Blisters:** Treat them with antiseptic. Watch for any changes or delay in healing and consult with your doctor if that happens.

✦ **If you get a cut or scratch**, treat it promptly. Wash the area in warm soapy water and use a mild antiseptic like Bactine. Cover the area with a dry sterile dressing and paper tape or a Telfa bandage. Don't use Band-Aids or adhesive tape. If the area turns red or swollen, or if there's any drainage, contact your doctor immediately.

✦ **If you get an infection**, do not walk or put weight on that area of your foot. Infections are like sponges. Putting pressure on an infection can spread fluids into other areas of the foot, thereby enlarging the area of the infection. Call your doctor immediately.

+ **Extremes**: Don't let your feet get too hot or too cold. Avoid sunburn, saunas and steam rooms, electric heating pads, or walking barefoot on hot pavement. Be extra protective of your feet in cold weather.
+ **Exercise**: Dr. Tim's diabetes educator recommends this gentle foot exercise—draw the letters of the alphabet with each foot every day.

your footwear

Buy leather shoes that provide protection by covering your feet completely. Your shoes should not be made of man-made materials because they do not breathe or stretch and may cause pressure on the bony areas of your feet. Look and feel inside your shoes each day. Shake out anything that may have lodged inside. Look at the soles for wear, or to see if you may have picked up a tack.

Your shoes should fit properly. There should be one-half to one finger of space between the end of the longest toe and the end of the shoe. The shoe width should be wide enough to accommodate the foot without pressure. Soles should be cushioned to absorb shock, and insoles should cushion the base of the foot. The arch of the shoe should support the arch of your foot. Feet grow and change, so shoe sizes must change accordingly.

Don't go barefoot. At the beach, wear sandals while walking on sand.

Wear a fresh pair of cotton or wool socks every day. If your feet perspire, change your socks several times each day. Does the top of your socks leave an indentation on your leg or ankle? If so, your circulation is being decreased or impaired. You can snip the tops of the socks with scissors or buy socks with larger tops. If there are marks on your feet where the seams make an indentation, wear your socks inside out or buy socks without seams. If you wear nylons, they should have a cotton sole.

Exercise your feet by walking daily. It helps improve the circulation to your lower limbs. After walking, check your feet for blisters or irritation.

A few more care ideas: take off your shoes and socks every time you see your doctor or diabetes educator. This will serve as a reminder to examine your feet.

And please, do not smoke. Smoking worsens blood flow to the feet. One cigarette a day constricts all your blood vessels for up to twenty-four hours. Blood vessel disease in the legs, feet, and hands is linked to smoking and tobacco use. If you want your feet to last a lifetime, quit smoking.

a new treatment

There is an especially promising treatment for diabetic peripheral neuropathy (DPN) called anodyne therapy that I read about in an article by diabetes educator Linda Hicks. When she first heard about it, she was skeptical and thought perhaps someone was trying to take advantage of those who suffer from DPN. Then she read that the FDA had cleared it as a treatment, so she tried it with six of her own patients. All six improved significantly. Pain levels were greatly reduced; they slept better and were able to go for walks again. Yet most doctors still believe that there is nothing that can be done for the pain of DPN.

Anodyne's effectiveness is based on findings of the 1998 Nobel Prize winner in Medicine. Nitric Oxide (NO) is a gas molecule and assists in the dilation of blood and lymph vessels. Excess sugar in the blood captures NO and stops it from doing its job effectively. Without sufficient NO, the capillaries can no longer provide nutrients and oxygen to the nerve cells, and pain and/or numbness results.

Anodyne uses small pads that emit infrared light and are placed lightly on the skin for forty-five minutes. The light energy releases the NO from its sugary prison so it can once more dilate the blood vessels. Because DPN is chronic, most people keep an Anodyne unit at home to maintain weekly treatments.

Until Anodyne, those suffering the pain of DPN had been told that there was nothing to do except take pain medication. Anodyne now offers real hope for relief. For information about this innovative treatment, call 800-521-6664 or go to www.anodynetherapy.com.

✦ ✦ ✦

your skin

Your skin is the largest organ in your body. It is your first responder against invading organisms. Poorly controlled diabetes affects the condition of your skin. It becomes more susceptible to dryness, caused by not enough fluids in the body. Bringing the blood sugar under control, drinking eight or more glasses of water a day, and using lotion containing lanolin can help dry skin. It's best to keep your skin soft and supple, so it doesn't crack and become a host for bacteria.

One skin problem specific to those with diabetes is called NLD—*necrobiosis lipiodica diabeticorum*. What a mouthful! Even though it's a relatively harmless condition, it can be quite disfiguring. It's believed that it results from an inflammation that destroys the layer of fat beneath the skin, leaving it dimpled and discolored. NLD occurs more frequently in women than men. It appears on the front of the legs as a shiny, tight, pink or red discoloration. NLD's danger is that the area may break open and become infected.

Acanthosis nigricans is a condition that is associated with insulin resistance. It appears as a thickening and darkening of the skin. It is sometimes a clue that someone may develop diabetes.

At present there aren't any medications that alleviate these problems, but they are helped by bringing blood sugar under good control and by reducing insulin resistance.

your immune system

Diabetes can affect your body's ability to heal. Your immune system defends your body by destroying bacteria and viruses. When blood sugar is elevated, the white blood cells in your immune system can't work effectively.

One white blood cell can destroy fourteen bacteria or viruses a minute. If a person eats six teaspoons of sugar (one donut or six ounces of soda pop), each white cell can only gobble up ten bacteria a minute for four to six hours. Eating twelve teaspoons of sugar (twelve ounces of soda pop or a piece of frosted chocolate cake) reduces that to only five bacteria per minute.

Eating eighteen teaspoons of sugar (cake with ice cream or a banana split), one white cell is only able to get rid of two bacteria or viruses.

The higher the amount of sugar in the blood, the less effective your immune system. When blood sugar is elevated, the body's ability to heal bites, injuries, infections, wounds, and skin ulcers becomes limited. It is not uncommon for people with consistent high blood sugar to complain of mosquito bites two months old that won't heal and razor nicks that won't close up.

Damage to small blood vessels causes poor blood flow to the skin. High blood sugar slows down the white blood cells so they can't fight bacteria and viruses. Together, these problems create a high level of risk for infections in people with diabetes. Infections may appear in the mouth, on the feet, in the bladder, in female genital organs, or any place there is a break in the skin.

Periodontal disease, cavities, and other mouth infections show up more often when diabetes is poorly controlled. Take good care of your teeth and gums by brushing and flossing your teeth at least two times a day, having your teeth cleaned and checked at least every six months, and reporting any "gum boils," loose teeth, mouth rashes, or sores to your dentist and doctor.

your brain

Insulin resistance is the primary cause of Type 2 diabetes. Obesity is the primary cause of insulin resistance. A recent study published in the *Proceedings of the National Academy of Science* showed that insulin resistance in the cells of the brain results in the same kind of changes that are seen in Alzheimer's disease. Dr. C. Ronald Kahn states, "This is the first clear demonstration of a biochemical link between insulin resistance and Alzheimer's disease, and it points to how understanding and developing new treatments for insulin resistance may have an impact not only in diabetes, but in many other common chronic diseases."

In a study of 6,370 individuals published in *Neurology*, there was a strong association between Type 2 diabetes and the onset of dementia in the elderly. Elderly patients with Type 2 had twice the risk of developing dementia or Alzheimer's as non-diabetic patients and those with Type 2 who were on insulin therapy had a four-fold risk.

your internal reality signal

I recently spoke to a friend who has written many popular books on living with diabetes. She told me of a man in his fifties who has two young children. Because of poorly controlled diabetes, he's lost his leg, several toes on the other foot, and is now blind. Barbara and the man's wife talked together recently. Upon learning of Barbara's long association with diabetes education, his wife sighed and said, "I wish he'd been willing to read a few of your books. We wouldn't be here right now."

Research is proceeding at an exhilarating pace. New treatments are being developed. Our understanding of the diabetes disease process is deepening each year. One theme keeps cropping up again and again: the closer to normal you keep your blood sugar levels, the better chance your body has to stay healthy. The severe complications of diabetes are often preventable.

We also know that for many people, Type 2 diabetes is preventable. The Diabetes Prevention Program (DPP) showed that people who are overweight and have impaired glucose tolerance (IGT) have a 50 percent chance of developing Type 2. By losing 7 percent of their body weight and walking twenty to thirty minutes a day for five days each week, people in the DPP cut their rate of progression from IGT to diabetes by 58 percent compared to those who took placebo pills. Those over sixty years old got an even bigger benefit: their progression to diabetes was 71 percent lower.

Many of us who have been involved with diabetes for a long time used to think of Type 2 diabetes as not as severe as Type 1, as a "sort-of" diabetes. We now know that whether you have Type 1 or Type 2, the complications are the same. Diabetes is your own personal IRS, Internal Reality Signal. If you don't pay attention to it now, it will get your attention later, but with fines and penalties added.

Being a hero means
meeting a challenge
with heart, mind,
and sinew.

chapter twelve

we all need a hero

S ome of these stories first appeared as articles in *The Diabetes Wellness Letter* published by the Diabetes Research and Wellness Foundation (DRWF). Mike Gretschel founded DRWF because he felt that not enough was being done to help people live with diabetes successfully. DRWF now sponsors diabetes seminars, offers phone counseling with a diabetes educator, and sends *The Diabetes Wellness Letter* to more than 50,000 people a month. In 1998, Mike asked me to interview people with diabetes and experts in diabetes care for the newsletter. Over the years, I have been privileged to talk with some extraordinary people who have met the challenge of diabetes with grace and courage.

Added to that are some good friends who, by their hard work and extraordinary service to others, continually inspire those with diabetes. I offer these stories to you to encourage you in your own journey.

✦ ✦ ✦

Steve Edelman

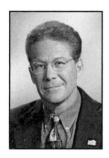

Dr. Steve Edelman is a Professor of Medicine at University of California at San Diego where he cares for patients and does research. He has a third full-time job as the volunteer founder and director of TCOYD, Taking Control of Your Diabetes.

Steve comes to his passion about diabetes education from his own personal experience. He was, as he says, a "chunky kid of fifteen" when he suddenly began to lose weight for no apparent reason. At first he was pleased, then symptoms like increased thirst and urination led his doctor to diagnose Type 1 diabetes.

He was in an HMO at the time and admits that for the first ten years he was under pretty poor control. Steve knew he wasn't following his diet plan, but his doctor didn't seem to notice.

"I'd get to the doctor's office early in the morning, (this was before the days of home glucose monitoring) give a blood and urine sample, and wait two or three hours for the results. Then the doctor would come in with a little clipboard, look at the numbers, and say, 'You're doing fine. I'll see you next time.'"

After years of this, Steve was smart enough to realize he wasn't doing that well. One hour before his doctor visit, he went to Winchell's and ate five donuts—two glazed, two chocolate cake, and one maple bar. Then he tested his urine. In about two seconds, the urine test strip turned dark blue, indicating very high blood sugar.

At the doctor's office, they drew blood and Steve waited an hour or so. The doctor came in, looked at his clipboard, looked Steve straight in the eye, and said "Steve, you're doing fine. I'll see you next time."

Steve's turning point had come. "I realized then that coming to him was a complete waste of time. He either didn't know or didn't care that my control was bad."

The good news was that he found a good doctor after that. The bad news was that he has some complications because of those first ten years of poor control. Steve says, "I have retinopathy, kidney disease, and neuropathy, but I ran into some good doctors in a timely manner so that I halted or slowed down the progression of the complications."

Steve decided to become a diabetes specialist and went to UCLA, got a master's degree, and then went on to medical school. It was as a physician specializing in diabetes that he realized that despite the publication of many studies that documented the benefits of tight control, diabetes care was not really getting any better.

Steve says, "I saw that despite new advances, new insulins, and home glucose monitoring, things were not improving at a community level. Not enough information was getting to patients. In 1995, I decided to put on my first patient conference called Taking Control of Your Diabetes at the San Diego Convention Center. We had over a thousand people, which is unheard of in patient education."

Steve feels that the most efficient and effective way to improve diabetes in this country is to get the information directly to the people who live with diabetes. And that's what he's doing.

He says, "It's not giving up on the doctors. Educate the doctors, yes, but educate the patients and their families in a parallel approach. Then create a free flow of information from the patient to the caregiver and back."

Since 1995, Steve and his staff have given conferences in twenty-five cities across the country. TCOYD is now a non-profit organization. They put on a one-day conference and health fair. They choose topics for those with Type 1 and Type 2, and for people caring for someone who has diabetes. Topics include blood pressure, heart disease, blood glucose monitoring, exercise, nutrition, and emotional issues. They have free foot exams and one-on-one sessions with exercise experts and diabetes educators. They always have a lawyer speak about legal issues, about the rights of those with diabetes and about how to manage "managed care."

TCOYD averages around 1,000 attendees at their conferences. They get the public's attention from many directions. They partner with national diabetes organizations, the AADE (American Association of Diabetes Educators) and primary care doctors in the area. They invite speakers from local hospitals and clinics who spread the word to their clients. TCOYD also has made connections with pharmacies, so that anytime someone picks up diabetes medication, they're given a flyer about an upcoming conference.

Steve notes, "It's not easy. It's a lot of work, but the rewards are worth it. We have so many testimonial letters, plus twice we've done a formal study about behavior in managing diabetes after the conference. We found that there was a marked result in people changing their behavior and taking control of their diabetes. One of the things we do is take away the fear and ignorance. Some people are so afraid of diabetes and the complications that it freezes them. It's the ostrich syndrome: they just put their head in the sand and hope nothing happens."

The other challenging aspect is funding the conferences. They cost about $150 per person, but each participant pays between $25 to $35. Companies and donors underwrite the balance. As Steve says, "We do a lot of begging from the pharmaceutical industry."

The best part for Steve is when people come up to speak with him at the conference and he sees that they are reinvigorated about controlling their diabetes. He says, "I look at my complications and I know they were preventable. If I can just help someone to understand his or her own history of diabetes, it can make a huge difference."

Steve started a free diabetes clinic in San Diego and publishes a quarterly newsletter. He knows the immense value of empowerment through education. He's also written a book titled *Taking Control of Your Diabetes*. You can check to see if a TCOYD seminar is coming to a city near you, become a member, and sign up for the newsletter at www.TCOYD.org or call 1-800-998-2693.

June Biermann and Barbara Toohey

June and Barbara are the authors of many highly regarded books about diabetes and are the founders of The Sugarfree Center in Los Angeles. The year I interviewed them, June had just celebrated her thirty-second anniversary of having diabetes and being complication-free by going to Hawaii. Early on, she decided to take charge of her diabetes; she set her own standards for blood sugar levels and for what she could and could not do. Diabetes has given her life, and Barbara's, an important focus— sharing their insights for successfully living with diabetes.

June was head librarian at Valley College when she found out about her diagnosis. She headed to the shelves around her for information. Every book she read sounded so grim, ". . . as if I'd have to spend the rest of my life as some kind of laboratory rat," she says. "I decided there must be a better way."

Barbara also worked at the library; in fact, June had hired her. They discovered their mutual love of writing and, by the time June's diabetes showed up, they'd written several books. Now they turned their attention to diabetes.

June says, "I was not about to reduce my image of myself to laboratory rat, but I could nestle up to the idea of guinea pig. I decided I was going to find out how best to care for myself."

Barbara convinced June to try skiing, even though at that time the popular wisdom held that a diabetic person shouldn't exercise. Soon June was at the ski resort, having just been put on injections and trying to balance food and insulin and exercise.

As June remembers, "Back then you didn't tell people you had diabetes. It was as if it were some kind of venereal disease." Yet she displayed her usual forthrightness and told the ski instructor that she was diabetic, just in case of an emergency. The ski instructor leaned in close and whispered, "So am I, but don't tell anyone or I could lose my job."

June found that skiing and diabetes worked together just fine, so she kept experimenting. She discovered a lot of things that were helpful in living with diabetes, but which didn't seem to be common knowledge. The next step was for her and Barbara to write about what they'd learned, but they weren't sure people would want to read about their adventures. Fortunately, their editor convinced them people would, and *The Peripatetic Diabetic* was published. They do thank their editor for the encouragement to write the book, but not for the title she chose. For years, they've been explaining that peripatetic means someone who gets around. Since then they've written many more books, "Fifteen if you count the rewrites and updates," Barbara says.

Another big venture was their homegrown "Sugarfree Center." It began as a mail order business out of their kitchen in 1978. They took a small ad in a diabetes magazine offering their books, a T-shirt, and a few diabetes items. From the responses, they realized that, as Barbara puts it, "People with diabetes in West Buffalo Breath, Wyoming couldn't get everything they needed to take care of themselves." Home blood glucose monitoring became available soon after and they began to stock essentials like Chemstrips and blood testing meters. Back then, Lifescan was just a small company in Britain and The Sugarfree Center was the first U.S. distributor for Lifescan's meters.

The business continued to grow, taking over a room above the garage. People in Los Angeles called and asked, "Since I live close by, can I come pick up my supplies in person?" A nurse was hired to demonstrate the proper use of the meters and answer questions. Then a dietitian. The business expanded to the house next door owned by Barbara's parents.

Then came the dreaded knock on the door. A man asked a simple question "Are you running a business in a residential neighborhood?" Presto, chango, they had two weeks to get the business out of the house. They found a location two blocks away and moved in, sharing the building with a few architects and contractors who loved to smoke and cuss. Not a perfect match. Fortune smiled, the rowdy guys moved out, and Barbara and June bought the building.

The Sugarfree Center was a wonderful place for me to go as the mother of a newly diagnosed child. The people who worked there really understood diabetes and its demands, and did their best to set your heart and mind at ease. Unfortunately, it no longer exists. From the original location they expanded to a second sight in Southern California and soon realized it was more than they wanted to handle. The business was bought by one company, then another. After that, Barbara and June moved on. But they couldn't "keep our paws off diabetes." They started the *Diabetic Reader*, a newsletter with the latest in diabetes info.

I asked these two seasoned diabetes experts for some sound advice on diabetes. They noted that for the parents of a diabetic child, the most important task is teaching the child self-care, taking responsibility in age-appropriate ways. For Type 1 folks, June says, "Know your numbers! You should know what your HbA1c level is, (the measure of your long-term blood sugar levels) your HDL and LDL, triglycerides, and cholesterol. Know the numbers and know what they mean. Don't accept a doctor telling you you're fine. It's your body and your health."

She says the same to Type 2 folks. "Don't accept a doctor saying you're doing fine. I don't understand doctors telling Type 2s to only test their blood sugar three times a week. That doesn't tell them very much. And I'm frustrated by this idea of having "borderline" diabetes, as many people call it. I wouldn't be surprised to hear that Type 2s have a larger statistical percentage of complications, because sometimes they've had it for years before it's diagnosed. The problems are sneaking up on them all that time. Also most Type 2s don't keep very close track of their blood sugar levels."

June and Barbara advise people to take diabetes seriously and "maybe it won't take you so seriously." June says, "With all the tools we now have to care for ourselves, there's good probability we can avoid complications and not feel we're the victims of cruel fate."

One view of June's life might be that "Cruel Fate" brought diabetes to her. The view I prefer is that it was good fortune that gave her a way to give so much to the rest of us.

Miss America 1999, Nicole Johnson

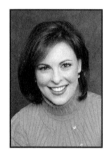

Several years ago I had the good fortune of teaming up with Miss America 1999, Nicole Johnson, for a number of diabetes-related events. Even if I hadn't met her, I would have remembered the night she was chosen, because my friend Deborah (from Virginia) called me, all excited.

"She won! Miss Virginia won!"

"That's wonderful, Deborah," I replied. "How great for Virginia."

"The heck with Virginia," Deborah retorted, "We're talking diabetes here."

I had forgotten that Miss Virginia was the young woman who had designated diabetes awareness as her platform, should she be crowned Miss America.

Once I'd met Nicole, there was no possibility of forgetting her or her mission. I was impressed by the strength of the conviction she conveys when she speaks. The words she uses are familiar, "don't let anyone stop you from following your goals and dreams" and "I'm grateful for each day," but their meaning is steeped in her getting diabetes at nineteen and what happened after that.

When she was first diagnosed, Nicole says, "I was devastated. I remember crying, wanting to know why. I thought I was dying. I didn't have a family history of diabetes and I had only been acquainted with one person who had diabetes, a high school classmate, and she had died. I thought that was happening to me. I thought my body was giving up and that it was all over. I lost a lot of self-esteem. I felt like I was damaged goods."

For Nicole, the road to recovering her sense of self lay in developing new skills. "As I learned to manage my diabetes, I saw that if I watched what I ate and if I exercised, I could keep it in control," she told me. "When I had good readings on my meter, I was like a child getting a good report card. It motivated me. But it took well over a year to get to the point where I accepted it and knew that I could have a normal life. I saw that I had to take complete responsibility, that it was in my hands. By that time, I was almost twenty-one and I decided to move into an apartment next to the university and live by myself."

Nicole also found, as many of us have, that reaching out to others as a volunteer or advocate helped her as much as it helped anybody else.

She volunteered to help with Juvenile Diabetes Research Foundation events in her hometown. She says, "I saw that I could make a difference in other people's lives. I had already gotten involved with competing in the Miss America program. This was four years ago. I graduated college and was working to get a master's degree in journalism."

Things were going along well. She was in graduate school and her diabetes was under control. One night, for no apparent reason, she became violently ill. The hospital called her parents and told them to get there immediately because "she's not going to make it." When her parents got there, they could barely recognize her. Her body was swollen and extremely toxic, her white blood cell count was almost nil, yet the doctors could not figure out what was wrong. Worst of all they would not allow her to take her insulin, nor would they allow her endocrinologist to see her. The bizarre aspect is that, in the midst of a life-threatening situation, the doctors were withholding the insulin that was essential to Nicole's life!

Fortunately, after much discussion, her parents took her home, even though she was still very ill. Home-care nurses came to see her every day. She was so weak that she could barely walk. Slowly she got better. No one ever figured out what was making her so sick, but she attributes her recovery to the power of prayer. Nicole has found that being close to losing her life helped her appreciate it all the more.

Her experience the first year she competed for Miss Virginia deepened her conviction to follow her goals and dreams. She was rooming with her chaperone and, "In the middle of the night, I somehow managed to fall onto her bed, even though I was in insulin shock. My pupils were dilated and I was not responsive. She called the paramedics. My blood sugar was so low, the meter could not even read it."

She had tried to hide her diabetes, afraid of what people would think, and now that wasn't possible. Nicole says, "Everyone in the pageant knew. I had had diabetes for four years, but it was only then that I decided that I had to genuinely accept it. I realized that having diabetes didn't make me a bad person, that other people's ideas about diabetes don't dictate who I am."

She had some advisors with the Miss Virginia pageant tell her not to come back next year, that there was no way they'd ever choose someone with a condition they'd have to worry about. They said, "Don't compete again. Don't do that to yourself. Don't do that to your family. You'll never go on to Miss America."

Nicole says, "I believed them for a little while and then I got angry. You don't give a type A person a challenge like that!"

She used the challenge to her advantage. She knew she'd never forgive herself if she gave up. She entered the local competition and won. She put together a public relations campaign for diabetes. She wanted people to understand that there was nothing wrong with her or anyone else who had diabetes. She appeared on television, did interviews, and wrote articles and posted them on the Internet.

"I'm thankful for the bad advice about not competing because that gave me the initiative to educate people about diabetes. I don't know that I ever would have been that motivated!"

In her interview for Miss Virginia she told them that "people have said that I can't do this, but I want you to know, I can. I wouldn't be here if I was incapable." After she won, several of the judges told her how impressed they were by her conviction. And that conviction carried her through to winning Miss America 1999.

This former Miss America, now known as Nicole Johnson Baker, has been very busy since relinquishing her crown. She and husband Scott recently welcomed little Ava Grace into the world. Nicole's become an important role model for people with diabetes, co-hosting the weekly CNBC diabetes talk show, *dLife*, and writing monthly columns for *Diabetes Health* magazine. She has had three books about diabetes published, with the fourth, *Mr. Food Diabetic Dinners in a Dash Featuring Nicole Johnson Baker*, to be released in March 2006 and a fifth, about her successful pregnancy, in the works.

Nicole feels that people with diabetes have to live more consciously and pay more attention. "Diabetes has changed the way I look at life. First of all, I view every day as a gift to me. Everyday that I wake up and feel good and don't have any complications, I know God has blessed me. I keep track of those days and am conscious of being thankful. If I have something that gets on my nerves, I step back and cool down. I realize that it's a small thing compared to the grand scheme of things. What's most important is life and secondly, what you choose to do with that life."

Gary Hall

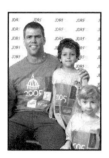

A few years ago, I watched as a swimmer named Gary Hall won an Olympic gold medal in Australia in the 50-meter free-style and which qualified him to be named "the world's fastest swimmer." He then went on to break a world record and win his second gold medal as a member of the U.S. 4x100 relay team. When the announcer mentioned that Gary had diabetes, I thought of what a great night that was for Gary and his family. Now that I've spoken with him, I have an even better sense of their joy.

Gary had been swimming competitively since age thirteen. It was in March of 1999 that he was told he had diabetes. He knew something was wrong, but wasn't sure what it was. There'd be times when his hands would shake uncontrollably and he'd have to leave a practice session to get something to eat. Then he got sick and wasn't getting better.

"Finally diabetes caught up with me. I was experiencing the symptoms, all of them: thirst and frequent urination, dizziness, blurred vision. I remember drinking two and a half gallons of orange juice in one sitting and I was still thirsty. It was at that point that I probably realized that there was something wrong."

When his doctor told Gary he had diabetes, it was a surprise because there was no family history. It was a disease that he didn't know anything about.

"I was devastated. One of my first questions was whether this was the end of my swimming career. The doctor's response wasn't very positive. He basically said it was unlikely I could continue, but I should get a second opinion. I was not only being handed the news that I had this disease that I was going to have to live with for the rest of my life, it was also like being told 'you're fired.' He told me this devastating information with one foot out the door. Then I went for a second opinion to an endocrinologist who told me that my swimming career was over, that I would never compete again."

Gary took a vacation. He decided he needed some time to figure out what he was going to do. He gathered together as much literature on diabetes as he could find and flew to Costa Rica. He spent a month and a half there, reading every day, educating himself about diabetes and how to manage it. He came back determined to find a new doctor.

"My father did some research while I was gone and located Dr. Ann Peters at the University of Southern California. I flew to Los Angeles and met with her. She was very encouraging. It made all the difference to me. She said she didn't see why I couldn't continue swimming. She flew up to Berkeley where I was training."

With Dr. Peters' help, Gary had a career-best time at the national championships just five months after being diagnosed. That's when he realized diabetes didn't have to stop him from competing. Gary proceeded, one goal at a time. First he made the Olympic team, then he began thinking that maybe he could win a gold medal.

Gary says, "When I was diagnosed, no sponsors would touch me. I couldn't get anyone to back me except for one vitamin company. It was a struggle and a gamble. I was $50,000 in debt when I went to the Olympics. Up until that moment when I won that race, I wasn't sure that it was going to work. It was very rewarding, not so much to prove the skeptics wrong, but I think, to inspire a lot of people with diabetes. And people who have not yet been diagnosed. When I was diagnosed there wasn't anybody that the endocrinologist knew to point to and say, 'Look, this guy has diabetes and he's managed it properly and he's managed to excel. He's even done better than before.' Nobody was there to say that to me at a very emotional time. Hopefully an example has been set for kids who want to be involved in sports. Not just kids, adults too."

Gary carries his One Touch glucose monitor with him, checking his blood sugar from four to ten times a day, depending on how his blood sugar is doing and if it's a day he's competing.

That night in Australia gave Gary a sense of accomplishment he will never forget. He hopes that a person with diabetes winning gold medals will broaden the public's mindset of what diabetes is and what a person with diabetes is capable of doing.

Gary says, "It's the cards you're dealt and you have to accept them. You make the best of it. The key is education and close monitoring. Take full advantage of the technology that has been afforded us. Use your blood sugar monitor and use it often. Pricking your finger four or five or six times a day seems like a nuisance, but it's nothing compared to losing your sight or your feet or the use of your kidneys. Diabetes doesn't have to be so much a disease as a condition. I think anything that's treatable and manageable can be looked at that way."

Gary sets an example that can be emulated: diabetes doesn't have to stop anyone from being a winner.

Dr. Francine Kaufman

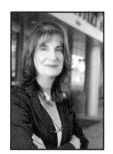

Childhood obesity is the cause of America's epidemic of Type 2 diabetes in children. Fortunately for all these children, Dr. Francine Kaufman is working on their behalf. When it comes to children and diabetes, there's no one more knowledgeable or passionate. Dr. Kaufman is a past president of the American Diabetes Association, Professor of Pediatrics at the Keck School of Medicine at the University of Southern California, and maintains a full-time practice at Children's Hospital of Los Angeles as the head of the Division of Endocrinology and Metabolism.

Her latest project is a study to understand how to treat Type 2 diabetes in children. She says, "When I started my career, maybe we had one child with Type 2. Now, at our center, at least 25 percent of the new cases are Type 2. That's one in four. Just about all of these children are obese. We're also seeing more chubby Type 1s, as the entire population gets heavier. If these children who are obese lose the weight and become fit, they probably will not have diabetes. We know that, early on, we can reverse Type 2 diabetes in children. Any weight loss accompanied by fitness improves blood sugar control. By fitness, I mean turning from completely sedentary to thirty minutes of walking five times a week. For a lot of these kids, if they lose weight and get fit a lot of the insulin resistance that is a factor in Type 2 diabetes goes away. The medication dose comes down, with better blood sugar control, better blood pressure, better everything."

She's observed that Type 2 diabetes in children is often a societal issue. Dr. Kaufman says, "I've been doing this for a long time and I'm amazed that there are whole pockets of our society that do not have access to the right information, who don't understand what a portion is, who don't understand how to read a food label. Once they're taught and given that information, they really do want to make the right health choices." Some families try to do what they know is right, but those who live in the poor areas of Los Angeles find that many grocery stores don't even carry fresh fruits and vegetables. (That really shocked me. I can't imagine feeding my children without access to fresh foods!) In some poor neighborhoods, there's no area to exercise. Dr. Kaufman said, "Those families feel doomed. And they are. Almost all of them try to make changes in the beginning, but the environment doesn't support a positive choice."

A lot can be done to support these families. Dr. Kaufman recently served on a White House "Summit on Healthy Schools/Healthy Students" and, as chair of a Blue Ribbon Task Force on fitness in children in Los Angeles County, led the effort to remove vending machines from school campuses across Los Angeles County. She notes, "We can also make an impact on the physical activity programs in our schools. Many schools have ditched them. The pressure is on to do well in standardized testing, and they don't have time for other courses. The dominant policy is, 'If I sit them at that desk long enough, they'll learn.' It doesn't even matter that it's the wrong kind of ideal. We need to do more about health and nutrition in the schools."

Dr. Kaufman has created a number of tools for managing diabetes, including insulin dosage guides and a CD-ROM diabetes game. She is also one of the medical directors of Camp Chinook, a camp for young people with diabetes in the San Bernardino Mountains.

Her many accomplishments have earned her the American Diabetes Association's Woman of Valor Award. Tommy Thompson, U.S. Secretary of Health & Human Services, presented it to her and noted that Dr. Kaufman "has the courage and drive to make a difference in the lives of millions, not just here, but around the world."

Allan Borgen

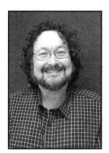

Allan Borgen has embarked on many career adventures and each of them has involved at least one of his two loves: food and children. His preferences began early. Allan says, "I grew up with a Jewish grandmother who did nothing but cook, cook, cook every day. She was from Europe and I asked her a lot of questions about food and culture and people. I was fascinated with how families in Europe ate. I've always had a love affair with food . . . and with children."

When he was sixteen, he began working at fast food restaurants. Then he graduated to the Hillcrest Country Club. Seven years later, Allan went through chef's training, but a year and a half into it decided the business end was not for him. Instead he got a master's degree in social work and worked for twenty-five years with abused and neglected children.

One day, he had lunch at a very good Chinese restaurant and enthusiastically told everyone at work about it. One of his co-workers said, "You're so passionate about it—you should do a restaurant guide."

Allan thought, "Why not?" He did some research and developed a restaurant guide. Then he had an idea for a television show. He approached the local PBS station and "nudged them for five months until they said yes." Fifteen years later, his restaurant review show, *Let's Dine Out,* reaches six to seven million Southern California homes.

Then Allan got Type 2 diabetes. "After so many years of making people fat, happy, and diabetic, including me, I decided it was time for some changes." This October, Allan welcomes a triple-threat co-host. She's a registered dietitian, a certified diabetes educator, and a fitness trainer. Besides reviewing mainstream food, they'll also be talking about what to eat that's diabetes friendly, low-carb friendly, and heart friendly.

Allan knows that some people learn more easily when they see something demonstrated, so he's working on a set of eight DVDs titled, *The Ultimate Guide to Diabetic Dining.* Allan says, "We'll cover Mexican, Chinese, Italian, fast food, and more. We'll show portion control and what to stay away from. We'll also include cooking demonstrations."

Recently, Allan's love of children and food has coalesced into a new mission. Allan kept seeing the same diabetic food products again and again, so four months ago, he opened the "Low-Carb, Sugar-Free Warehouse." The store carries an amazing array of foods for those on restricted diets. A third of his customers have diabetes. This new retail venture has put Allan in touch with many newly diagnosed children and their parents. They've inspired Allan to create a DVD just for them, titled *You're Not Alone.*

Allan says, "The worst thing is to feel you're alone and there's no help. As a social worker and as a person with diabetes, I'm familiar with all the feelings that come up. That's my new role in life, instead of making people fat and happy, it's to make them healthy and happy."

The enthusiasm and insight of the children and parents who took part in the filming of the DVD impressed Allan. He says, "The parents shared how devastated they were when they were told their children had diabetes. The kids were so open and honest. What I got from the kids was 'Don't give up.' Don't let your friends influence you. Be positive."

On the DVD one eleven year-old girl named Sarah calmly told how some of her friends said they didn't want to play with her because they would catch diabetes. Then she burst into tears. Everyone in the studio cried with her. Several teens advised her that at first they didn't want to tell their friends, because they were afraid that they'd be an outcast, but they learned as they got older to tell people about it. They've learned to talk with their peers and their teachers about what they need.

Some of the children expressed frustration with the daily unpredictability of trying to control blood sugar levels. They said that even when they try to eat the same thing at the same meal and monitor their levels, the results are different every day. Siblings told of their feelings of responsibility. Gabrielle, Sarah's sister, admitted she feels she should watch Sarah and help her be okay. One thirteen-year-old teen spoke of how he helps his newly diagnosed sister cope. Some children told of going to Grandma and Grandpa's house and being offered candy and ice cream, making it hard for them to stay within their food plan.

"Diabetes affects the whole family. Everyone needs to be involved in supporting the demands of diabetes. Helping children and families with diabetes is now an obsession for me. Whatever I can do for them is my new mission." Allan says.

Allan is very excited about another DVD he recently completed, *The Ultimate Guide to Diabetic Foot Care*. It presents recommended guidelines for proper diabetic foot care with practical demonstrations that are easy to understand. According to the U.S. National Diabetes Advisory Board, "Early detection and appropriate treatment of foot ulcers may prevent up to 85 percent of foot amputations." To order a copy of Allan's DVDs, visit: www.e3resourcemedia.com or call 1-800-691-3035.

Dr. Ann Peters Harmel

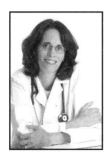

As a child, Dr. Ann Peters Harmel loved science and loved people, so when she grew up, it was quite natural for her to become a doctor. At a recent event to raise money for stem cell research, she told me, "I found I was really interested in diseases that affected the mind and body. I learned very early on that not only was diabetes a disease that most doctors didn't want to treat because it required a long-term connection with patients, but it also was a mind-body disease. I've pursued my entire career taking care of people with diabetes and loving it."

Her specialty is caring for pregnant women who have diabetes. She's very good at it. She is the director of clinical diabetes programs at the University of Southern California and runs two diabetes clinics. One is near Beverly Hills. The other is the Roybal Comprehensive Diabetes Program in East Los Angeles where she cares for patients who don't have health insurance. She said, "I see the richest and the poorest people in Los Angeles. I'm also involved in the countywide effort to provide diabetes care for people who don't have health insurance. Rich, poor, and in-between, I want everybody to have good medical care."

Through her experience and the research she's done, she's learned that she can teach people how to use their medicine and how to test their blood sugar, but that doesn't equal good control. Good control comes from having a health care team that supports you, not just your doctors, but also your family and your friends. She has seen that success is most often dependent on having people who help you get motivated to take better care of yourself.

Controlling diabetes is always a challenge, and pregnancy only adds to that challenge. It used to be that if you were a young woman with diabetes, you would most likely be told not to have children. Because blood sugar control was not as finely tuned as it is now, the risk of damage to the baby and the mother was very high. Now we know that women with diabetes can have healthy babies. Home blood glucose monitoring has allowed people with diabetes to follow intensive insulin regimens, which can achieve blood sugar control very close to that of a person without diabetes.

Dr. Peters Harmel told me, "When you have diabetes, the risk of problems in the baby is always a little higher because glucose is never completely normal. I do invite women to have as close to a normal hemoglobin A1c as possible before they conceive. That's an A1c less than 7, but most of my patients already have that."

A successful pregnancy with diabetes is completely possible, but the caveat is if there are too many preexisting complications. If a woman already has kidney disease, heart disease, or eye disease, it may not be possible. Every woman who is contemplating pregnancy needs to see an eye doctor. Dr. Peters Harmel says, "I don't care if they have to drive 1000 miles. They need to make sure their eyes are okay, because retinopathy can worsen during pregnancy." She also recommends that the doctor test blood pressure and kidney function, so if there's any issue, they can be on blood pressure medicines. If there's any heart disease, that also needs to be addressed before pregnancy.

Dr. Peters Harmel adds, "Short of that, I take care of all sorts of women who do beautifully through their pregnancy. I've never had a bad outcome. We have lots of healthy moms and babies in our practice."

In addition to blood testing, the insulin pump has also positively affected pregnancy with diabetes. Many of her patients choose to be on the insulin pump, because they can't use Lantus, as it hasn't yet been approved for use during pregnancy. She notes, "A lot of my patients are on Lantus with pre-meal injections of a rapid-acting like Novolog or Humalog, but when they're anticipating pregnancy, they go off the Lantus and most go onto the pump. Very few go back on NPH."

The growth of the baby changes the need for insulin. Early in pregnancy, blood sugar levels go down, so less insulin may be needed. As the pregnancy progresses and the placenta grows, it causes insulin resistance. Blood sugar levels rise, requiring more insulin. Dr. Peters Harmel recommends that pregnant diabetic women check in with their health care team every week to address what's happening with their insulin requirements. Then when the baby is born, the insulin requirements go way down. She says, "If it's your first pregnancy, you won't know these things. That's why those of us who've cared for hundreds of women through pregnancy understand what is needed."

She recommends that women who are considering pregnancy take extra folate (folic acid). Her team gives nutrition counseling and believes that good nutrition should be largely the same prior to pregnancy, during pregnancy, and after pregnancy, with the addition of folate supplementation and getting adequate calcium.

Ensuring the health of diabetic moms and their babies is a very specialized field. There's almost no challenge Dr. Peters Harmel and her team hasn't seen. Plus, as she says, "We're all moms, so we know what it's like to have a baby, breast-feed, and not get any sleep. We've been through it. I think it's that support that makes it possible for our patients to do so well."

✦ ✦ ✦

John McDonough

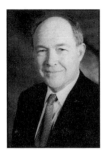

John McDonough is mostly retired now, having served as CEO of Newell Rubbermaid and Chairman of the Board of the Juvenile Diabetes Research Foundation. John got diabetes when he was six years old.

"In those days, sixty years ago, the doctors told my parents that I would live until I was fifteen or maybe twenty. That was what they expected. My paternal grandfather died of diabetes in the late 1920s about the time insulin became available. My mother, who was really tough, would talk with me about that, that I might only live a few more years. I finally got to the point where I wasn't afraid of dying so much as not living."

These beliefs about diabetes colored John's approach to life. "I was a lousy diabetic teenager. I thought, 'What do I have to lose?' Then I met my future wife Marilyn and I saw that I had everything to lose. She told me to clean up my act or get out of her life."

Marilyn adds, "I met John when I was fifteen. I had an aunt who died in a diabetic coma and my father was very upset that I was going out with John." John cleaned up his act, love prevailed, and they've been married for more than forty-five years.

After getting married, John forged ahead with his life, infused with a sense of urgency. "You spend your life in a hurry. You've got to make money, take care of your wife and children. You've got to get all these things done. I understood at twenty, instead of at forty, that this isn't a dress rehearsal."

The biggest challenge for John was the way other people looked at him. He remembers, "When I was a kid in grade school, kids (who knew he had diabetes) would make fun of me. Somebody would say something to me and I wouldn't say a word—I'd just start swinging. When I got married and had kids, I couldn't get life insurance. I once was with a company and they talked about my becoming the president. The CEO took the position that I wasn't going to be around that long, so I didn't get it. That was in the 1970s. The statistics said that you wouldn't live very long if you had diabetes."

How did John feel about that? His response, "Oh, I just got mad and I've stayed mad all my life," is punctuated by a full-blown belly laugh.

With the help and support of his wife Marilyn, John has taken good care of himself. He's had good reasons to do so. One was that he enjoyed building his business and he knew that he couldn't work that hard if he didn't feel well. His daughter Allison is his other good reason. She got diabetes more than twenty years ago.

Sixty plus years of diabetes has taken a toll: part of John's leg. He handled it with his usual McDonough initiative and wit. John remembers how it all started. "I was always careful with my feet, because I knew the risks. Nonetheless, I developed an infection. We tried everything, but it just wouldn't heal. First I lost one toe, then a second. I was in the hospital a lot, on all kinds of medications, plus antibiotics."

One night Marilyn noticed a long red streak extending from the infected area up his leg. John had had an aortic valve replaced in his heart and they both knew if that long red streak of infection reached that valve, it could be deadly. Over the course of the next thirty-five days, John had ten surgeries. He lost his leg below the knee. John says, "It took me a while to come back. I had a fever for a long time and the wound wouldn't heal. They opened it up again and put packing in it every day. There was pain, let me tell you— yelling, screaming pain. Finally they were able to close it up."

During this whole time, his daughter Allison stayed with him to help manage his diabetes. "She slept on a naugahyde chair every night," John says, "For Christmas that year I offered to buy her a naugahyde chair of her very own." John notes that her response is unrepeatable in polite company.

The hospital recommended that John be fitted with a prosthesis. It was not a good experience. The shop was dingy looking. There wasn't any parking close by, and he and Allison had to park half a block away. John says, "It was awful. Allison started to cry, saying 'Oh, Dad, after all you've been through, now this.' I assured her there was one good thing. 'I'll only worry about athlete's foot half as much as I used to.' She started laughing and then we both did. That helped us get through that day."

John fell down the first time he tried to stand on the prothesis, but eventually he got better with it, even though walking was difficult and uncomfortable. Legendary baseball player Ron Santo had been a friend of

John's for many years and Ron lost both his legs to diabetes. John says, "He and I became really close when he was going through it. Ron introduced me to a new prosthesis technology and it made a huge difference."

The technology is called the Harmony System and it addresses the fact that fluid volume in the leg changes. Fluid volume is most stable at night during sleep, but during the day, it can change from 7 to 12 percent causing the limb to be a different size and shape. When you get up in the morning, the leg is at its largest volume and as the day progresses, it decreases. A conventional prosthesis is fitted for only one volume, so if it's fitted early in the day, it might fit well in the morning, but may be too loose in the afternoon as the limb volume decreases. Conversely, if the prosthesis is fitted in the afternoon, when fluids are less and the leg is slightly smaller, it may be too tight in the morning. Either method of fitting a conventional prosthesis may result in an uncomfortable fit during the day. The rubbing on the end of the limb can cause pain and subsequent irritation and breakdown.

A below-knee amputee and prosthetist, Carl Caspers invented the Harmony System. The prosthesis contains a pump that stabilizes leg volume and maintains proper fit throughout the day. It also helps to reduce perspiration. Ray McKinney assisted Carl by field testing the technology and providing valuable patient feedback that helped improve the system.

John says, "This leg has changed my life. I put it on in the morning and don't take it off until bedtime. Ron is out riding his horse and playing golf. He has two of them: one leg is blue and one is white. He says they're his 'home and away' legs." (Relating to the Chicago Cubs' baseball uniforms.)

Ron and John were so impressed they bought the technology and created McKinney Prosthetics in Gurnee, Illinois. John says, "We're helping a lot of people. The shop is clean, bright, and welcoming. We even serve coffee. I wanted going into that shop to be part of the healing process."

The cost of the Harmony System can be several thousands of dollars. It is incorporated into the prosthesis and is designed to fit each individual. Insurance companies recognize the technology and its benefits, and cover a substantial portion of the cost. Although John's company has been able to help some people who can't afford their system, they can't do as much as they would like.

John says, "We see so many people who need help. Right now there's a young woman who lost both legs to cancer and she can't afford our legs. So

we started a new foundation, 'Limbs for Life,' to help those who need it."
John has other plans, too. Right now, there's only the one shop near Chicago,
but plans are in place to open satellite offices around the country. Perhaps
someday everyone who has a prosthesis will feel the way John does, "This
leg is only an inconvenience."

Carol and Erwin Lurie

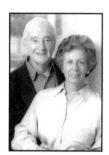 Stephen Lurie, son of Carol and Erwin, was diagnosed
with diabetes in 1970. Thus began an exceptional journey
of commitment and perseverance.

Carol's grandmother had diabetes, but Carol felt
completely unprepared for her son's diagnosis and for
how much there was to learn. She recalls, "Back then
there wasn't any home blood testing. We did urine
tests, using a second void. Do you know what it takes to get a little boy
of ten to give you a second void of urine? And then, what do you do after
you've found the doctor, after you've learned how to give insulin injections,
after you've become the nurse at home, the caregiver?"

If you're Carol and Erwin, you look around to see who understands what
you're going through. You look for someone who is doing something to help.
Carol says, "We joined one organization, but there was very little effort going
toward research." The Luries wanted more; they wanted a cure for their son.

Two months after Stephen was diagnosed, they heard about a convention
in Miami Beach for a new organization to fund research. Erwin and Carol
flew to Florida to attend what they thought was a big convention, walked into
the meeting room, and met twenty other parents of diabetic children. They
also met the woman from Philadelphia who had arranged the convention.

That extraordinary woman is Lee Ducat, whose young son Larry had
been diagnosed with diabetes. Lee felt that existing diabetes organizations
were not sufficiently focused on research, so she created a new organization
named the Juvenile Diabetes Foundation, devoted solely to finding a cure
for diabetes and its complications. (A few years ago, the name was expanded
to Juvenile Diabetes Research Foundation.)

Carol's admiration for Lee is absolute. "If ever there was a woman who can make up her mind and accomplish what she wants to do, it's Lee Ducat. She taught us how to get to a senator, even to the president. She never took 'no' for an answer. She was the mentor, the mother of JDRF."

Inspired by Lee's example, the Luries were determined to spread the word. Carol says, "When we got home, Erwin and I established the New York Chapter. The first year we were in business, we did an event at the Starlight Roof of the Waldorf Astoria Hotel. Erwin had to underwrite the event personally because we had no credibility, no track record. And then we sold out!"

After that, wherever Erwin went on business, he helped organize a JDF chapter. In Chicago, Erwin invited two diabetes groups who'd been working independently to a meeting. Then he locked the door and told them, "You're not getting out of here tonight until you join together and create one chapter, plus elect a president, a vice-president of fundraising, and a finance volunteer." They did.

JDRF's volunteers became aware that no matter how much money they raised, they needed the involvement of the U.S. government and its resources in the search for a cure. So Lee and Carol went to Washington, D.C. Carol remembers, "Lee and I had an appointment at the White House. As they walked up the driveway, I looked up at heaven and said, 'Oh, if my mother could only see me now!'"

Carol has many extraordinary memories of her years with JDRF. While they were on a cruise to the Far East, word reached them that there was a shortage of insulin in China. They called Novo Nordisk, who generously arranged for one hundred vials of insulin to be waiting for them at the next port. It was brought onto the ship and safely stored in the captain's refrigerator.

Then they received a message that the Chinese authorities had contacted the captain. They knew about the insulin onboard and assumed that Carol and Erwin were going to sell it on the black market. They were ready to confiscate the insulin and the Luries!

Intense conversations with interpreters were held, letters from the children's hospital in Beijing presented, and all was smoothed over. Even so, Carol didn't feel at ease until the insulin was delivered. She said, "I couldn't have been happier when we got it to the hospital. The hugs and kisses we received from nurses and doctors made it all worthwhile."

A few years ago, after so many years of fundraising and chapter building, Carol thought it was time to retire, but then her grandchild was diagnosed. She says, "Everything you've worked so hard for has to start all over again. You stay onboard."

Fundraising for diabetes research is a family affair. Carol's older son Jim, who does not have diabetes, sits on JDRF's International Board as VP of Finance. Carol says, "I have so much respect for this organization. I've watched it grow. Without all the people who have given of themselves to find a cure, we wouldn't be where we are today, respected throughout the world. One perk of being a part of this organization is being able to pick up the phone and speak to any researcher in the world. All you have to tell them is you're part of the Juvenile Diabetes Research Foundation and they take your call."

Carol and Erwin's first event in New York raised $10,000. Thirty-five years later, the New York chapter raises over $10 million a year. This year, JRDF International has pledged $100 million to diabetes research, continuing its reputation as the largest private supporter of diabetes research in the world. (Only the U.S. government spends more and that, too, has been influenced by the many years JDRF volunteers have spent on Capitol Hill.) It all began with Lee Ducat, Carol and Erwin Lurie, and twenty people in a room in Miami Beach.

As we were completing our conversation, I asked Carol, "How's your son, Stephen?"

She said, "I'm very blessed. Stephen is doing very well. That was as of yesterday at about two in the afternoon. I hope and pray that continues."

Dr. Michael Brownlee

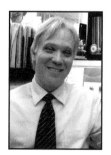

Michael Brownlee's life epitomizes his favorite quote from T. S. Eliot's *Four Quartets*, "We shall not cease from exploration, and the end of all our exploring will be to arrive where we started and know the place for the first time."

Although his exploring days are far from finished, Michael Brownlee has reached a peak that permits him a moment of reflection. He was recently awarded the American Diabetes

Association's highest research award, The Frederick Banting Medal, making him only the third active diabetes researcher in the world to achieve the "Triple Crown" of diabetes research awards, which includes the European Association for the Study of Diabetes' Claude Bernard Medal and the ADA's Outstanding Scientific Achievement Award. He is the senior author of a comprehensive chapter on all aspects of diabetic complications in the latest edition of *Williams Textbook of Endocrinology*, considered the gold standard in the field. He holds the Anita and Jack Saltz Chair of Diabetes Research at the Albert Einstein College of Medicine, where he is a Professor of Medicine and Pathology and co-founder of its Diabetes Research Center. He is the leader of an international center for the study of diabetic complications funded by the Juvenile Diabetes Research Foundation.

Michael's journey with diabetes began almost fifty years ago, when he was diagnosed with Type 1 at the age of eight.

He remembers, "At that time, the medical profession believed that diabetes caused metabolic effects like high blood sugar and high blood fats, and also damaged your blood vessels and nerves. The thinking was that there was no connection between high blood sugar and the damage, that those were independent effects of diabetes. Based on that thinking, the prevailing view was that you should keep out of ketoacidosis and avoid severe low blood sugar, which also can cause coma and death. Otherwise you could do what you want and blood sugar didn't really matter."

However, there was another viewpoint at the Joslin Clinic in Boston, one of the world leaders in research and diabetes care. Michael says, "They didn't have a lot of data, but they approached it from a logical point of view. Their argument was that if the body were designed so that the blood sugar shouldn't vary too much, there must be a good reason. Therefore, if your blood sugar was above normal, that's not natural and it couldn't be good."

Fortunately for Michael's long-term health, his parents adopted the Joslin approach of balancing food and insulin in a very precise way. It wasn't easy: Every bit of his food was weighed on a gram scale, and at that time, there was no technology for people with diabetes to measure and monitor their own blood sugar levels.

Michael wanted to study medicine. He didn't know how many obstacles would be put in his path. While attending college, he worked one summer in the clinical chemistry lab at the Washington, D.C. Veterans Administration Hospital. Since he was very efficient, they asked him to help write papers. He recalls, "I was allowed into the inner sanctum, the medical library. There I discovered the *Williams Textbook of Endocrinology*, which opened up a whole new world for me. That was the first time I had ever read all the really terrible details about diabetic complications. Up until then I had had only a vague notion of what they were and what caused them, but here were all the disturbing statistics in front of me."

Those statistics included the warning that a person with Type 1 diabetes could be assured of living into his thirties at most. That might have discouraged some, but not Michael. He continued with his dreams, and decided to dedicate his life to finding new drugs that could prevent and treat diabetic complications. When he applied to medical schools, several told him outright that their policy was not to take "people like you," because they felt that after educating him, he was going to die early and it didn't make much sense. Undaunted, he contacted various diabetes experts and asked them who they thought was doing interesting research. One of them was Rubin Bressler, a Canadian who had had diabetes since he was three, and was a professor at Duke University. Michael contacted him and was invited to a meeting.

"We hit it off right away," Michael says. "We talked about his exciting research and by the end of the day, he said he was going to write a letter about me to the admissions committee and that's how I got into medical school."

Before beginning medical school, Michael went to a recommended diabetes doctor to have a physical exam. After examining him, the doctor told Michael he had hemorrhages in his eyes.

Michael recalls, "That stunned me, because to a lay person, the word hemorrhage means major bleeding, but he was actually referring to some tiny little red dots in my retina. I learned then that how doctors talk to patients, and understanding what the patient is thinking and feeling are very important."

Michael sought out another specialist who "knew I was a struggling medical student and said he'd make a deal with me. He said he'd take care of me and he wouldn't charge me if I would promise to do the same for others when I was in his position. And I have."

His first exam results showed he had protein in his urine, signaling possible kidney failure. His new doctor reassured him that mistakes could be made.

He was right: there was a mistake and Michael's kidneys were fine. Even so, the experience had shaken Michael so much that he decided to finish medical school in three years instead of four. And he met that goal, while, at the same time, putting in a year of laboratory research.

During medical school, he often used himself as a guinea pig. Michael arranged for a friend to come over on Sunday and put an IV in Michael's arm with a constant rate of glucose infusion. Then Michael would take an injection of Regular insulin, drink lots of water, and test his urine for sugar every hour. Using the urine volume and glucose concentration, he figured out the grams of sugar that were spilling out in his urine. Knowing how much sugar was going in per hour through the IV and how much was coming out in his urine helped him calculate how long the insulin was lasting and how effective it was. He was able to create an insulin program for himself that mimicked the way insulin pumps work today.

Michael did his residency at Stanford and began his investigation of diabetes and its complications at Harvard Medical School and the Joslin Diabetes Center. He then began sharing his newly researched perspective with the medical community and was invited to a debate in front of a group of pediatric endocrinologists, who were outraged by the idea of such meticulous care. Michael says, "They attacked me. They said, 'You don't understand the first thing about children and their psychosocial development. You would ruin these children for any kind of a life.' They were so angry. Now pediatricians are the strongest advocates of self-monitoring of blood glucose, tight control, and insulin pumps. Medical progress has often been like that."

The last few years have been especially rewarding for him. Professionally, he has discovered the unifying mechanism underlying diabetic complications, and is hard at work designing novel therapeutics for preventing and treating diabetic complications. The pace of research progress constantly excites him. He is now the author of the chapter in *Williams Textbook* that he first read so long ago. Personally, he enjoys good health and is free from complications, and enjoys the company of the love of his life, Karen.

Michael has beaten the odds. He feels certain he is still healthy because of his parents choosing the Joslin approach to diabetes care all those years ago. He says, "Knowing the statistics I read in the *Williams Textbook* in my first year of college, I never thought I'd be alive to write a chapter as a senior contributor. Nobody's been more surprised than I have about just being here."

Receiving the award named for Frederick Banting, who discovered insulin, also has a personal meaning because, as Michael says, "Without Frederick Banting, I would have died when I was eight years old."

His whole-hearted enthusiasm for diabetes research continues. Michael says, "There was a long period of time when the ability of research was limited by a lot of technical barriers that were insurmountable, but that's all gone now. We've discovered the way all the complications fit together, how they relate to each other. It's very exciting to see that out of that model have come three first-generation drugs. When these things work, it really is an incredible rush for me."

Knowing the damage diabetes can do has been a burden. He notes, "You lose the gift of being ignorant. You can't fool yourself into believing, 'Well, if this happens, I can do this or do that.' My wife Karen has taught me how to fully appreciate living each day. When I first met her, I thought 'There must be something wrong here. Nobody can be so completely happy and in love with life.' But she is! She's filled my life with a grace and a joy that has displaced all that heavy feeling of 'who knows what's going to happen around the corner.' I wake up in the morning and say, 'I'm so grateful for another day.'"

Dr. Michael Brownlee knows that he and all people with diabetes stand on the shoulders of the diabetes researchers who went before. He clearly sees the long road he has traveled from first confronting the personal and scientific problems of diabetic complications, to now, where he knows so much more about both. He has arrived where he started, supported and challenged by the work of Frederick Banting and the authors of that old edition of *Williams Textbook*. And, with a refreshed sense of purpose, he understands his journey as if "for the first time."

There are so many more people I could include. There's my friend Mark Blatstein, who didn't let being fifty years old (with forty years of diabetes under his belt) stop him from competing in a world-class competition in tae kwon do. There's my friend Deborah who made the decision when she was diagnosed at nine to never let diabetes stop her from having a great life. She knew to be free to live her life as she wished she would have to take meticulous care of her diabetes, and she has. Her A1c readings are regularly below 6.

There's thirty-six-year-old Will Cross, who has Type 1 diabetes. He's set a goal to be the first person with diabetes to climb the highest mountains on the world's seven continents as part of the NovoLog *Ultimate Walk to Cure Diabetes*, the "Peaks and Poles Challenge." He's already completed a successful mission to the South Pole and North Pole, and ascended Argentina's 22,840 foot Mount Aconcagua and Alaska's Denali at 20,320 feet. He still has Russia's Mount Elbrus, Antarctica's Mount Vinson, the Carstenz Pyramid in Indonesia, Tanzania's Mount Kilimanjaro, and the world's highest peak, Mount Everest to go. And he intends to complete all these climbs within two years.

The accomplishments of these people are founded on perspective and commitment. Each set a goal and did not give up. For them, "No" or "You can't do that" were not acceptable answers. They are heroes, yes, but no more a hero than you can be to your family and friends.

Being a hero means meeting a challenge with heart, mind, and sinew. It means moving forward in spite of fear. It means getting to the end of our days and being able to say, "I did the very best I could." It means leaving a legacy of effort and grace to our loved ones. And it is the greatest gift we can give.

dr. tim answers
frequently asked questions

Why me? Why did I have to get diabetes?

Your diabetes may be the result of your genetic heritage, but most likely it's the outcome of choices you've made. Diabetes occurs in the rich and poor, young and old and it's most often a lifestyle disease. It's the result of inactivity coupled with eating too much food. The extra weight gained creates insulin resistance.

Some people who maintain normal weight and activity levels do get Type 2, but the number is small compared to the total number of people with Type 2 in North America. In some cases, diabetes developed after a prescription for high doses of prednisone, a steroid used to treat certain medical problems.

All of the patients we treat with Type 2 diabetes are overweight. Changing your lifestyle will help control the disease. A frequently heard saying is that if you keep doing what you have been doing, you will get the same result. Make a change.

I've just been diagnosed with type 2. Do I need insulin?

The answer is yes, you do need insulin, but you may not need insulin injections. Type 2 diabetes is a deficiency of insulin or a resistance to the body using the insulin that you are making. The result is the same: not enough insulin. Often oral medications can sufficiently decrease your blood sugar.

There are four types of oral diabetes medications and each type can decrease your blood sugar between 30 and 60 points. Someday you may need insulin, either by injection or in the form of insulin spray (available soon). Type 2 diabetes is a deficiency of insulin, so taking insulin helps you feel better and have more energy. Insulin also has no limit to the amount it can decrease your blood sugar, as compared to oral medications. Of course, nobody likes shots, but my patients do like the results the injections provide. Sometimes there's fear surrounding the idea of sticking yourself with a needle. That's when you need the support of an expert. One of my patients, a nine-year-old girl who's had diabetes for four years, taught a newly diagnosed forty-year old woman that she could give herself a shot that didn't hurt. If the time comes for you to need insulin injections, it will help to have the support of someone who's an "old hand" at it, along with your diabetes team.

I have type 2 diabetes. Will my spouse develop it too?

Diabetes isn't contagious, so why do so many husbands and wives both have Type 2 diabetes? The medical term is "associative mating." People tend to marry someone of similar physical appearance and lifestyle habits like smoking, drinking and dietary habits. Since Type 2 diabetes is related to lifestyle, your spouse is more likely to develop Type 2 diabetes than your friends are. The upside to this is that being married to someone with a chronic disease can improve your health. How? It's called the "spin-off effect." It's seen in men who have a heart attack and begin an exercise program in a cardiac rehabilitation program. Spouses are often welcome to participate in these programs free of charge. It's been observed that as the health of the heart attack survivor improves, the health of the spouse also improves.

I imagine that you and your spouse eat in the same restaurants and eat similar foods at home. We live in a food-crazed environment. We had lunch today at a restaurant that featured a new dessert: a deep-fried Twinkie covered with chocolate and served with ice cream. Yuck! I can't think of anything that better demonstrates how many bad food choices there are. We have to take our health back one day at a time. Every restaurant, every meal offers us both healthy and unhealthy food choices. Every day offers you both a chance to get moving and maintain your health through appropriate exercise. The good thing is that you can support and encourage each other and then share the rewards of good health.

I believe in treating problems naturally. How can I avoid taking drugs?

The most helpful, natural thing you can do is to lose enough weight to be at your ideal weight and add exercise. A quick formula for determining your ideal weight is: Women should weigh 100 pounds for five feet tall. For each inch over five feet, add 5 pounds. Therefore, a 5'5" female should weigh 100 + 5" x 5 = 125 pounds.

A man should weigh 106 pounds for five feet tall plus 6 pounds for each additional inch of height. Therefore a 5'10" male should weigh 106 + 10 x 6 =166. These weights seem low because they are ideal weights based on longevity. At a lower weight, your pancreas is able to produce less insulin and its function can be preserved. Exercise also helps to control diabetes since glucose uptake by the muscles can occur without extra insulin being secreted.

There are trace minerals that can be helpful. One, vanadium in the form of vanadyl, can cause decreases in weight, glucose levels, triglycerides, and cholesterol as it helps decrease cravings and total food intake. Vanadyl helps to lower blood sugar if you have diabetes, but doesn't lower blood sugar if you don't have diabetes. Take a maximum of 25 mg daily, but if you have kidney problems, don't take any. Vanadium-rich foods include chocolate, kelp, mushrooms, dairy products, and seafood.

Magnesium may be helpful and have a protective effect on preventing diabetes from developing. Magnesium-rich foods include peanuts, tofu, broccoli, and nuts and seeds. Foods high in magnesium may be better tolerated than magnesium supplements as some forms of magnesium such as Milk of Magnesia may cause loose stools.

Chromium is the third trace mineral. It's also called the glucose tolerance factor. At the Joslin Diabetes Center, large doses of the trace element were used to lower blood sugar and cholesterol levels. Higher doses decrease blood sugar more quickly, but by four months, a dose as low as 200 micrograms worked as well as a dose of 1000 micrograms. Foods that are high in chromium are meat, whole grains, oysters, cheese, and brewers yeast. The best-tolerated form is chromium polynicotinate, followed by chromium picolinate. Ask your health care provider if these trace minerals are right for you.

Recently, the journal *Diabetes* printed an article showing that cinnamon in small amounts can help control blood glucose. In the study by Alam Kahn, Ph.D., in Pakistan, sixty men and women with Type 2 diabetes were given different doses of cinnamon. The doses were 1/4 teaspoon, less than 1 teaspoon, and 1 3/4 teaspoon. Twenty days after stopping the cinnamon, there was an 18 percent to 29 percent reduction in blood sugar levels. The reduction continued in those taking 1/4 tsp. doses. Cinnamon was also effective in lowering triglycerides at the 1 3/4 tsp. dose level.

Lowering your blood glucose an average of 30 points in a month can decrease your HbA1c by 1 percent. This is dramatic and is a treatment that is certainly easy to swallow. Each decrease in HbA1c of 1 percent lowers your risk of diabetes complications by 35 percent.

My uncle had his feet amputated because of diabetes. Could that happen to me?

The wife of one of my patients, Hal, recently gave her husband a picture of a man from a magazine. While he was watching, she took out a scissors and cut off the legs of the man in the picture. Hal asked what she was doing. She said, "Hal, I'm tired of trying to get you out of your recliner. This will be you in ten years if you don't make a change in your life."

Hal's wife got his attention that day. He came to the office for our diabetes education program. He had a cardiac treadmill test and started an exercise program.

What happened to your uncle doesn't have to happen to you. Good blood glucose control, plus exercise, attentive foot care, and comfortable, padded shoes can help you keep your feet for a lifetime. If you are having any foot problems, ask your physician for a referral to a foot specialist.

What's the formula for calculating my average blood glucose level for the past three months?

A useful approach to determine your blood glucose control is to use your HbA1c, the blood test that measures your average glucose levels for the past ninety days. Higher than normal blood sugar causes proteins to bind to the hemoglobin and decreases the amount of oxygen available to your tissues. Normal HbA1c is 5.3. At this level, 5.3 percent of your blood will not be carrying oxygen. At 5.4, your body will start developing inflammation of the arteries and begin setting the stage for heart disease.

The formula is HbA1c - 2= ___ X 30= average blood glucose for 3 months.

For example, an HbA1c of 7.0 translates to 7 - 2 = 5 X 30 = 150 average blood glucose.

The American Diabetes Association recommends an HbA1c below 7.0 while the American College of Endocrinologists recommends an HbA1c of 6.5. Because vascular inflammation begins to occur when the HbA1c is above 5.4, lower is better unless you are having too many problems with hypoglycemic reactions.

Will I be able to keep my job now that I have diabetes?

That depends on the conditions of your employment. One patient of mine, Danny, faced that question recently. He's a trucker and had been diagnosed with Type 2 diabetes, but didn't worry about it or treat it aggressively. He was in the office for a truck driver exam and we found that he had significant neuropathy in his feet. Danny was taking maximum doses of oral diabetes medications, but wouldn't agree to take insulin because his company prohibits driving a truck if insulin is used.

Danny admitted that he couldn't feel the accelerator pedal or brake so would look to see if his foot was on the correct pedal. It's scary to think of an 80,000 pound truck controlled by someone who can't feel his feet. Danny's truck driving days were over, but the position of dispatcher became available and he accepted. Although he can work, he can't drive a car or truck so his wife drives him to work. The system made it difficult for Danny to both control his diabetes properly and work as a truck driver.

Jim, who works at the post office, had a coworker recently say to him, "I don't know how much longer I can keep working because I've been diagnosed with diabetes." Jim was surprised: he had continued working for several years after being diagnosed with diabetes and never gave a thought to stopping. He'd been able to take good care of his feet also, as postal employees have access to great shoes that are not available to the general public. Jim's coworker was delighted to hear that he could work as long as he took care of his blood glucose and cared for his feet.

Why can't I lose weight?

I frequently hear from patients, "When I was a teenager I was determined that I wouldn't gain weight like my relatives." So what happens?

It happens gradually. Children, work, hobbies all begin to take time that could be devoted to leisure or exercise. Then add in quick meals on the run, sitting at children's sport practices and events, and snacking to keep awake to accomplish one more activity and you start gaining weight.

Many people are like Patti who has Type 2 diabetes and decided she was going to exercise to lose weight, but didn't change her eating patterns very much. After a month of weightlifting, walking, and biking, she'd gained five pounds. She gave up. Sound familiar?

There's Faith Sommers, who did succeed. She went from wearing baggy clothes to hide excess weight to being proud of her body. She says, "One day I was really feeling down and tried to recall the last time I'd felt good about myself. I drew a blank. I decided it was time for a change. I substituted turkey sandwiches and salads for fast foods, ate pretzels or fruit in place of chips and cookies, and drank at least eight glasses of water daily.

"Then I added exercise. I went to the gym daily at 6:00 A.M. That time was a big struggle for me. I walked 30 minutes on a treadmill and eventually ran 3 miles per session. After 2 months I lost 15 pounds and people encouraged me. A year later I'd lost 60 pounds and hit a plateau. I decided to vary my exercise program and increased running time each week. It took 2 years to lose 105 pounds. One of the best moments of my life was wearing a two-piece swimsuit at the beach. I felt so confident. My workout schedule of weight training 3 times a week, then biking or walking 45 minutes 3 times weekly had paid off. I wish I had lost weight sooner, because I love my new life."

Shape magazine has a monthly success article about a woman who has lost weight and kept it off. The one common denominator in all the weight loss stories is that the women exercised 7-10 hours a week, and limited fats and carbohydrates.

How can I avoid having to go on dialysis?

Damage to the small blood vessels in the kidneys occurs in Type 2 diabetes about the same time as you develop diabetic changes in your eyes. Since you've probably had diabetes for 5-10 years before you were diagnosed, your kidneys may have been affected, especially if you have had higher than normal blood sugars and/or high blood pressure.

If you have Type 2 diabetes, then ask for a urine microalbumin test. If you are spilling microalbumin in the urine, then you need immediate treatment. If you smoke, *stop*. Everything about diabetes is made worse by smoking. What do you ask for if you have microalbumin in the urine? Ask for aggressive treatment for blood pressure, ACE inhibitor medications, or ARBs (angiotensin receptor blockers). Both classes of medication help your kidneys and have few side effects. Maintain near normal blood sugar and eat a low-protein diet.

I've just been diagnosed with diabetes and have heard that it causes blindness. How?

The lens in your eye is very sensitive to changes in blood sugar levels. High blood sugar causes the lens to change shape, resulting in blurred vision. This usually improves as the levels are closer to normal, but can last a few weeks, if your blood sugar fluctuates widely and is uncontrolled. Cataracts can develop at a younger age and new growth of capillaries can occur. Small aneurysms can develop in the arteries in the back of your eye. If the aneurysm breaks, then bleeding occurs in the eye and affects your vision.

At early stages, these problems are treatable. Since you may have had diabetes for 5-10 years before you were diagnosed, it's essential that you see an eye care specialist as soon as possible. New treatments can help maintain your vision for a lifetime. Most insurance companies pay for diabetes eye exams, because they know that preventing complications will save your vision and save them money. Ask your healthcare provider for a referral to an eye care specialist for an annual diabetes eye exam.

First we're told to lower our fat intake. Then we're told that fats are good for us. I'm confused!

In our frenzy to avoid fat, many of us have not learned that there are fats that heal. Fats that occur naturally in many foods can heal us by decreasing inflammation in our heart arteries. "Essential" fats are fats that the body needs to thrive. If you don't include these in your diet, you will be more likely to have a degenerative disease, such as arthritis, diabetes, coronary artery disease, or cancer.

If you were born in the year 2000, you will have a 50 percent chance of having cancer in your lifetime. It's time to give your children and grandchildren a better chance for health by understanding the role of "good" fats.

Essential fatty acids (EFA) are healthy fats. Their names are linoleic acid and alpha linolenic acid. These fats attract oxygen. EFAs are involved in producing life energy in our body from substances and moving the energy throughout the body. They govern growth, vitality, and mental state. EFAs transfer oxygen throughout thin membranes in the lungs, in capillary walls, and in the walls of red blood cells to hemoglobin that is carried to every cell in the body. EFAs are part of all cell membranes. We need a 4 to 1 to 1 ratio of omega 3s, to omega 6s, to omega 9s.

Omega 3 rich foods include salmon, trout, mackerel, sardines, flax, canola oil, soy, walnuts, and dark green leafy vegetables. Eating fish twice weekly can significantly decrease your risk for heart disease. Omega 6 rich foods include most seeds, safflower, sunflower, soybean, walnut, evening primrose oil, and meats. Omega 9 rich foods include most nuts: almond, peanut, pistachio, pecan, canola, avocado, hazelnut, cashew, and macadamia nuts and meats. Type 2 diabetes causes inflammation of the arteries and these EFAs can reduce inflammation in the arteries. Eating a few nuts daily can also reduce your risk for heart disease.

One pill for blood sugar, two for blood pressure, another for high cholesterol, aspirin for inflammation. My cupboard is starting to look like my grandparents' house. How can I get rid of some of these medications?

There is no doubt that we live better through chemistry with antibiotics and medications to treat myriad medical problems. Some people hate taking medications. So what can you do? It's possible you can take fewer or reduced amounts of some medication if you make a few lifestyle changes.

Work with your healthcare provider to develop an exercise program. Exercise allows the body to lower blood sugar with less medication or, in some cases, no medication. Blood pressure can improve with loss of body fat, but can't always be controlled without medication. LDL cholesterol, the culprit for depositing plaque in your arteries, can be greatly reduced with weight loss, exercise, and by taking soluble fiber with meals. Two teaspoonfuls of freshly ground flaxseed with meals will often lower LDL cholesterol. Your goal with LDL is to keep the level below 100. If you need to take statin medications like Lipitor, Pravachol, Zocor, Mevacor, or Lescol, there is an upside. These medications decrease the risk of stroke and heart attacks and some studies show they help prevent Alzheimer's disease. If your cholesterol is normal and you take a statin medication, it decreases your risk for heart disease even more. Change what you can and accept what you can't change.

How can I increase my HDL cholesterol?

Everyone should know his or her HDL cholesterol level. HDL is sometimes called the vacuum cleaner of your arteries. Less than 5 percent of people know their HDL and ignorance can be costly. "Raising HDL may be more important than lowering LDL cholesterol," says Daniel Rader, Director of Preventive Cardiology at the University of Pennsylvania School of Medicine. Ideal HDL should be greater than 50 for women and greater than 40 for men. A new treatment with injectible HDL cholesterol can decrease plaque in the arteries by 4 percent in three weeks. Until the new treatment is available, here are a few ways to increase your HDL:

1. Quitting smoking increases HDL 11 percent
2. Losing weight helps.
3. Replace margarine or butter with olive oil or Benecol.
4. Aerobic exercise increases HDL 13 percent
5. Alcohol raises HDL, but doctors urge moderation.
6. Statin medications raise HDL 5-6 percent.
7. Fibrates like Tricor or Lopid can increase HDL by 10-20 percent.
8. Niacin, a B vitamin, can increase HDL by 15-30 percent.
   It does have some side effects: flushing, itching and tingling skin.

Regarding the side effects: Niaspan, the prescription form of niacin, causes less flushing and itching, but is more expensive. Take it at night and you can sleep through the side effects! If you take aspirin, then take it before the niacin to blunt the side effects and avoid acid foods prior to taking the niacin since they increase flushing. Acid foods include coffee, soda pop, spicy foods, and orange juice. Niacinamide does not work for HDL. Avoid the use of sustained-release, over-the-counter niacin as it is hard on the liver. Niaspan is an extended release formula that does not cause the liver problems associated with sustained-release products.

Should I worry about my child's cholesterol?

High cholesterol has been a concern of those forty years old and up, but research published in the *Journal of the American Medical Association* shows that high cholesterol in the teen years predicts dangerous thickening of the artery walls in adulthood. The American Academy of Pediatrics recommends cholesterol screening for kids who have a family history of heart disease, who have a parent with high cholesterol, or for those whose parents' medical histories aren't known.

You should foster a heart-healthy diet and regular exercise regimen for your child. Have the pediatrician check his cholesterol once he's in his teens. The acceptable level for anyone under nineteen years of age is 170. Any number over 200 is considered high. Studies of 2,600 people who had high cholesterol as teenagers and then were tested as adults showed a much greater chance of plaque buildup. Overweight teens, those that smoked or had high blood pressure had similar plaque buildup. Medications like Lipitor lower cholesterol, but most doctors don't use these in teenagers because of concerns about liver toxicity. Limiting saturated fat to 10% of the daily intake can help.

What can I do if I have the "metabolic syndrome"?

Twenty-five percent of Americans have this problem and it's increasing. In the metabolic syndrome, your body makes insulin, but the cells do not allow all of the insulin to enter the cells, so the insulin is at high levels in the blood vessels and causes all types of changes. High insulin levels cause vascular inflammation, fat production, and an increase in triglycerides, blood pressure, and waist size. This combination leads to vascular inflammation and higher risk of heart attacks.

The best treatment is reversing what caused the metabolic syndrome in the first place. Exercise is the key. How much? Start a walking program and increase it slowly. Work up to walking an hour every day, or try 5 minutes of exercise 12 times per day, or 10 minutes 6 times per day. Just start moving again!

Metformin, also known as Glucophage, can reduce the metabolic syndrome. It is the only medication that helps weight loss. Actos and Avandia can cause weight gain while they are correcting the metabolic problems. When you take any of these medications then your energy increases as glucose gets into your cells and you feel like doing more activities. Ask your healthcare provider about treatment for the metabolic syndrome, but start walking. Every little bit of exercise helps.

How can I lower my cholesterol level?

We need cholesterol to live as it is used to make hormones that regulate our bodies. The problem arises when the bad cholesterol increases and aids in blocking arteries of the heart, brain, or legs.

New recommendations are for LDL ("bad") cholesterol levels to be less than 100. Many cardiologists are trying to achieve lower levels to prevent or treat heart disease. Your choices concerning diet and exercise will make a dramatic difference, but only 1 in 3 people are able to decrease their LDL cholesterol to less than 100 without medication.

If you can't get your LDL below 100 with lifestyle changes, statin medications can cause dramatic decreases in LDL cholesterol. When combined with Zetia, a newer medication that binds LDL in the bowel, LDL goals below 100 can be achieved. A warning: in a small percentage of people, statins can cause liver damage, muscle aches, and joint pains so you will need to be monitored by your healthcare provider. Statins most often used are Lipitor, Zocor, Pravachol, Mevacor, and now Crestor. A generic statin, Lovastatin, is now available. The statin medications also decrease inflammation in the arteries. Why is this important? Half of the people that have a heart attack have normal cholesterol. In these cases, inflammation is the culprit.

I'm in menopause and I've just been diagnosed with diabetes. Help!

Type 2 diabetes causes enough changes in your life without adding menopause to the mix. Menopause is the curve ball thrown just when you think things are settling down. Your children have finished school. You are already enjoying grandchildren. You have some free time on your hands, then puberty happens in reverse. Hot flashes, mood changes, and sexual problems. And that's just the beginning for some women!

Your metabolism slows down and body fat increases. Fat produces some estrogen, so maybe you have fewer hot flashes, but the fat increases insulin resistance. Dry eyes and vaginal membranes become annoying. Vaginal yeast infections are more common and your body changes the bad cholesterol from normal-size LDL particles to small, dense LDL particles that act like termites and burrow into the walls of your arteries. The signs and symptoms of menopause are due to unreliable estrogen levels.

What helps? Herbs can help, but may take three months to begin working. Soy at 4-7 grams per day decreases total cholesterol and triglycerides. Black cohosh 40-80 mg two times daily and Red Clover-Promensil slightly decrease hot flashes. Exercise will help decrease insulin resistance and high blood glucose. Avoid spicy foods as they increase hot flashes. Wear light clothes to bed. For hot flashes, The American Association of Diabetes Educators recommends sub-therapeutic levels of SSRI medications. These selective serotonin re-uptake inhibitors help stabilize your serotonin levels and help mood changes. The doses are lower than the doses used to treat depression. Effexor 37.5 mg or Prozac 10 mg may work within two weeks.

Estrogen reverses signs and symptoms of menopause but because of concern about increased breast or uterine cancers, this needs to be discussed with your health care provider. Prescription Clonidine patches can decrease hot flashes, but you may need a high dose and if it's stopped abruptly, it can cause severe high blood pressure.

✦ ✦ ✦

Should I have a cat scan of my heart?

In non-diabetic people, research has shown a distinct relationship between coronary artery calcium buildup and the amount of plaque in the heart arteries. CAT scanning of the heart has been shown to predict future coronary events, such as heart attack. If a person doesn't have diabetes, the amount of calcium in their arteries is related to their risk of heart attack

Many X-ray centers now offer coronary CAT Scans, which is useful in non-diabetic people, but it is not a reliable predictor of heart attacks in those who have diabetes. This may seem confusing as people with Type 2 diabetes have a high number of coronary problems. Even though people with Type 2 diabetes generally have more calcium in their arteries, a direct relationship between the amount of calcium and heart attack risk has not been established. Coronary events are due to rupture of plaque and not from plaque build-up only. Diabetes alters plaque to make it less stable, therefore more vulnerable to rupture. If you have Type 2 diabetes, you are better off treating your lipids, blood pressure, and blood sugars, and exercising and taking aspirin as recommended by your healthcare provider.

What are trans fats?

To make it simple, trans fats are fats that have added hydrogen, which makes them solid at room temperature. The problem is that the fats are chemically changed so that your body cannot process them. Foods high in trans fats are pastries, chips, cookies, French fries, many brands of margarine, Crisco, and peanut butter that doesn't require stirring. Read the labels and look for "hydrogenated oil" of any kind. Don't buy or eat that product.

What can you eat? Fruit, vegetables, low-fat cheeses, and whole-grain crackers. Look for labels that say, "No trans fats." "I Can't Believe It's Not Butter" is low in trans fats. Low-fat yogurt, fresh bean dip, and hummus are trans fat free. Use olive or canola oil for cooking and eat fish twice weekly. And cut way back on fast foods, or "window foods," as a friend calls them.

Is my child at risk for developing type 2 diabetes?

Type 2 diabetes was once thought to be associated with middle age, but as our children have become overweight and less active, Type 2 has reached epidemic levels in American children.

Carlos is an example. He was diagnosed with Type 2 when he was sixteen years old. He was never a good enough player to make a high school sport team, but he excelled at video games and spent hours on the computer and watching TV. Carlos had most of the risk factors for Type 2 diabetes: he is Hispanic, spent 4-6 hours on the computer and watched television daily, and had a family history of diabetes. He developed fatigue, blurred vision, weight gain, and dark pigmentation around his neck. Carlos took medications to lower blood sugar, but sixteen years ago diabetic management teams were rare and Carlos had no such help.

By the time he was thirty-two, he developed chest pain and was diagnosed with angina, a decreased blood supply to the heart, a disease usually associated with middle age. Carlos had a stent (tube) placed in the narrowed coronary artery. It keeps the blood flowing while he's in cardiac rehabilitation. They take him through a daily exercise program and a lifestyle program to restore health.

To prevent Type 2 diabetes in your child, cut back on the risk factors you can control. Limit television and computer time to one hour a day, unless it's for schoolwork. Encourage regular physical activity and sports. Limit your child's intake of soda pop, sports drinks, and juices, and have him drink more water. Also limit fast foods to only once a week. To learn more, you can call 1-800-342-2383 or go to www.diabetes.org.

Is the south beach diet good for people with diabetes?

I think it can be. To me, the South Beach Diet is more like an IQ test to see if you can apply healthy eating principles. It was designed for people who feel like their life is ruled by food cravings. The goal of the program is to avoid heart and vascular disease by eating healthy fats and healthy carbohydrates. You'll lose weight as a byproduct. The author, Dr. Arthur Agatston, M.D., used this program for his patients to avoid blocked arteries and the inflammation of the blocked vessels

Insulin resistance, the cause of most Type 2 diabetes, is an impairment of insulin's ability to properly process fuel, the fats and sugars. As a result, the body stores too much fat, especially belly fat. Much of our weight gain comes from carbohydrates, especially the highly processed ones in baked goods, breads, snacks, and packaged desserts. The goal is to increase fiber-rich carbohydrates while curtailing the bad carbs, the highly processed ones where all the fiber has been stripped away. Eat more fruits, vegetables, and whole grains. Avoid carbohydrates made with white or enriched flour as most of the nutrients have been removed and only a few nutrients have been added back.

Lean beef, pork, and lamb are permitted. Chicken, turkey, fish, nuts, low-fat cheeses, and yogurt are permitted. Low-fat food other than dairy products can be fattening. Oils from olive and peanut and canola (rapeseed) are allowed as they reduce the risk of heart attack and stroke.

How do I give my sore fingers a break?

Several meters allow your fingers a rest from pokes for blood tests. Our certified diabetes educator, Yvonne Ferguson, RN, has been delighted with the "Freestyle" meter which allows you to test on the forearm, upper arm, thigh, calf, or hand for variety. New Accucheck meters also allow alternate site testing. You may be limited to the meter that's paid for by your insurance company, but ask at the pharmacy to see what's new in glucose monitors that will simplify your life. You can then contact your insurance company and see if they'll cover one of the newer models. A caveat: if you think your blood sugar is low, then test on your fingertips because other areas of the body are less sensitive to rapid changes in blood glucose.

My husband falls asleep while driving the car. When he drives off the road into the gravel he wakes up, but he won't let me drive! What can I do?

The question above came from a sixty-five-year-old woman whose husband (who has Type 2) "snores like a train coming through a tunnel and stops breathing for several seconds several times at night." Sleep apnea is more common in Type 2 diabetes, because of the associated weight gain. As we gain weight, structures in the neck and around the airway become thicker. During sleep, the tongue falls backward and the airway is reduced in size.

During sleep, your mind and body recuperate. What if you don't sleep well? Tomorrow you may think less clearly, you may get sleepy even on short drives and you'll wonder where your zest for life went. Poor sleep causes insulin resistance that can result in Type 2 diabetes. Lack of sleep also causes stress hormones to be released including adrenaline that raise blood sugar levels.

State law required that I report Jean's husband to the DMV. He participated in a sleep study and it showed that he awakened over one hundred times at night, but he wasn't awake enough to be aware of it. With a C-PAP positive airway pressure mask to wear at night, Jean's husband is now able to sleep like a baby and stay awake all day.

Snoring from A to ZZZZ is a book by Derek Lipman, M.D., an ear, nose, and throat specialist in Portland, Oregon. If there is a loved one in your life who snores loudly and has episodes of stopped breathing at night, then ask for a sleep study. You may save a life.

resources for readers

To order Gloria Loring's relaxation CD,
Body, Breath, & Mind,
go to www.glorialoring.com

American Association of Diabetes Educators
100 West Monroe Street, Suite 400
Chicago, Il 60603
Phone 800-338-3633
www.aadenet.org

American Diabetes Association
National Call Center
1701 North Beauregard Street
Alexandria, VA, 22311
www.diabetes.org

Canadian Diabetes Association
Association Canadienne du Diabete
www.diabetes.ca

Children with Diabetes
www.childrenwithdiabetes.com

Diabetic Cooking magazine
P.O. Box 505
Mt. Morris, IL 61054-0505
800-777-5582

Diabetes Exercise and Sports Association
P.O. Box 1935
Litchfield Park. AZ 85340
800-898-4322
www.diabetes-exercise.org

Diabetes Forecast magazine
A healthy living magazine from the ADA
1-800-DIABETES (1-800-342-2383)
www.diabetes.org

Diabetes United Kingdom
www.diabetes.org.uk

Diabetes Research and Wellness Foundation
P.O. Box 96046
Washington, D.C. 20077-7240T
www.diabeteswellness.net
To subscribe to the *Diabetes Wellness News*
Call 866-293-3155

International Diabetes Federation
Avenue Emile De Mot 19, B-100
Brussels, Belgium
Phone 32 2 538 5511
www.idf.org

Joslin Diabetes Center
The World's Leading Diabetes Center
One Joslin Place
Boston, MA 02215
1-617-732-4000
www.joslin.org

Juvenile Diabetes Research Foundation
Dedicated to finding a cure for diabetes.
120 Wall Street
New York, NY 1005-4001
Phone 800-533-2873
www.jdrf.org

Milner-Fenwick, Inc. Diabetes Educational Videos
2125 Greenspring Drive
Timonium, MD 21093-3113
www.milner-fenwick.com

National Diabetes Information Clearinghouse
Diabetes Prevention Program
1 Information Way
Bethesda, MD 20892-3560
ndic@info.niddk.nih.gov

National Institute of Health
Part of the National Diabetes Education Program
More than 50 ways to prevent diabetes.
1-800-439-5383
www.ndep.nih.gov then search "50 ways"

TCOYD—Take Charge of Your Diabetes
Available in English, Spanish and Braille
1-877-232-3422
www.cdc.gov/diabetes

"What is your risk for developing diabetes?
Tests you can take online for diabetes and all of the
degenerative diseases.
www.yourdiseaserisk.harvard.edu

diabetes exam recommendations

Make copies of this page and take to every visit with your doctor to remind you of what you and your doctor can discuss.

once a year:

✦   *Urine microalbumin*—Your goal is below 30. It checks for protein in the urine, an early sign of kidney disease.

✦   *Comprehensive foot exam* to check circulation, nerves, and skin to prevent long-term damage and amputations.

✦   *Flu vaccine* every autumn to help prevent influenza.

✦   *Dilated eye examination* to check for eye damage from diabetes.

✦   *Self-management goals*—Discuss how you can set goals for controlling your diabetes.

every 3 to 6 months:

✦   *HbA1c*—The goal is below 7.0. (Below 6.5 is even better.) It measures the control of your blood glucose for the past 2-3 months.

✦   *LDL cholesterol*—Below 100. (Below 70 is even better.)

✦   *A brief foot exam and blood pressure test*—A goal of 130/80 is ideal to help prevent kidney damage, heart attacks, and strokes.

✦   *Aspirin* is recommended in people over the age of 40 with diabetes. Talk to your doctor.

✦   *ACE or ARB* use if you have high blood pressure or protein in the urine.

✦   One more: Get at least one *pneumonia vaccine* in your lifetime. Repeat every 5 years in most individuals. These help prevent common types of pneumonia, meningitis, and sepsis (overwhelming infections).

blood glucose monitors

To help you choose a blood glucose monitor, talk with your diabetes educator or doctor and ask other people with diabetes what they are using.

Also, consider purchasing a unit at your local pharmacy. Your pharmacist has chosen the meters based on reliability and ease of use. Purchase locally even if you mail order your subsequent diabetes supplies. The convenience of having a local pharmacist to discuss diabetes issues with is invaluable and your local pharmacy will carry lancets, test strips, and batteries for your unit. Following is a list of several of the major companies' web sites and phone numbers, and the blood glucose monitors they offer

Abbott Laboratories ✦ www.medisense.com 1-800-527-3339

1. **Precision QID.**
   This unit allows you up to 30 seconds to get enough of a blood sample to test.

2. **Precision Xtra.**
   The monitor is backlit and provides you with data management. It also tests for ketones, so is more useful for Type 1 diabetes.

3. **Precision Softact.**
   It was one of the first monitors to provide alternate site testing.

4. **Freestyle Flash.**
   Multiple site testing is encouraged and a data cable is available to upload your blood glucose records.

5. **Freestyle Tracker.**
   Blood glucose monitor plus a PDA plus a carbohydrate value food list with hundreds of foods listed on it.

Bayer Diagnostics ✦ www.bayerdiag.com/products 914-631-8000

1. **Ascensia Breeze.**
   It provides blood underfill detection, saves up to 100 tests, and is downloadable.

2. **Ascensia Contour.**
   It allows multiple site testing, the information is downloadable, and the results are available in 15 seconds.

3. **Ascensia Dex 2.**
   It provides multiple site testing and it codes itself automatically. The autodisc loads 10 tests at one time. With its 100-test memory and downloadable features, it is popular.

4. **Ascensia Elite.**
   It is simple to use, there are no buttons, and it allows multiple site testing.

5. **Ascensia Elite Xl.**
   The unit turns on when a test strip is inserted. It allows multiple site testing, saves up to 120 tests, and is downloadable.

Becton, Dickinson, and Co. ✦ www.bddiabetes.com 1-888-BDCARES

1. **BD Logic.**
   This unit stores up to 250 tests results and contains software that is downloadable. It also keeps records of the insulin you have used.

Home Diagnostics Inc. ✦ www.prestigesmartsystem.com
1-888-777-7357

1. **Prestige IQ.**
   The unit allows uploading to the internet, averaging of results every 2 or 4 weeks, and works in the range of 25 to 600 blood glucose range.

2. **Truetrack Smart System.**
   This unit requires a very small sample of blood, it has an audible test strip fill detection, and allows alternate site testing.

Hypoguard ✦ www.hypoguard.com 1-800-818-8877

1. **Assure Hypoguard.** This unit eliminates the need for cleaning and a code chip is included in each box of strips. It stores 180 tests and software is available.

2. **Assure II Hypoguard.** This is similar to the Hypoguard and it has an automatic "on" feature when a test strip is inserted.

3. **Assure III.** This unit works in 10 seconds and does not require cleaning.

4. **Advance Micro-draw.** Very little blood is required for testing; it saves 250 tests and is downloadable.

Lifescan ✦ www.LifeScan.com 1-800-227-8862

1. **One Touch Basic.**
   This monitor works in several languages. It saves dates and times and holds 75 tests in memory.

2. **Induo.**

   This unit tests in five seconds and also contains insulin for convenience in one unit. It notes when the insulin injection has been given and records the date of the most recent dosage.

3. **One Touch Surestep.**

   The unit gives results within 15 seconds, it averages for two weeks and one month, and is downloadable.

4. **One Touch Ultra.**

   The unit allows multiple site testing with results in five seconds.

5. **One Touch Ultrasmart.**

   Alternate site testing and five-second results make this unit useful. Its PDA-like face allows information about exercise, food, medications, and comments to be made and shows patterns on the screen.

Roche Diagnostics ✦ www.accuchek.com 1-800-858-8072

1. **Accu-chek Active.**

   The unit provides results in five seconds and allows multiple site testing.

2. **Accu-check Advantage.**

   The popularity of this unit is due to its comfort curve test strip that fits the shape of the finger.

3. **Accu-check Compact.**

   Self-contained strips are held on a drum, eight second testing, and a small sample of blood make this a popular choice.

✦   ✦   ✦

4. **Accu-check Complete.**
   The unit contains graphs and charts to follow your progress and it uses the comfort curve test strips.

5. **Accu-check Voicemate.**
   This unit allows users with low vision to test by prompting to simplify use. The comfort curve test strips are also used.

Wal-Mart ✦ www.wsff.com/relion/index.html 1-888-922-0400

1. **Relion Ultima.**
   No wiping or cleaning is necessary and the unit has a memory for 450 test results.

GLORIA LORING is one of the most versatile singers of her generation, and has been described by *Los Angeles Times* critic Don Heckman as having "one of the best vocal instruments in pop music since the salad days of Barbra Streisand." Her career has spanned more than three decades of recordings, concert tours, and appearances on stage, television, and radio. She is also a songwriter and co-composer of television theme songs for *Diff'rent Strokes* and *Facts of Life*, and starred as "Liz Chandler" on NBC's *Days of Our Lives* for six and a half years. Gloria is well known as a spokesperson for the Juvenile Diabetes Research Foundation. When her son was diagnosed with diabetes at age four, she created and self-published two volumes of the Days of Our Lives *Celebrity Cookbook* to raise money for diabetes research. Those books, along with her recording *A Shot in the Dark*, raised more than one million dollars for diabetes research. She followed that success with two more commercially published books, *Kids, Food, and Diabetes*, and *Parenting a Child with Diabetes*. Currently she writes a column for the *Diabetes Wellness Letter* published by the Diabetes Research and Wellness Foundation.

On the lecture circuit, Gloria Loring presents a musical-motivational seminar: *Turn the Page*. Combining biographical anecdotes, personal growth insight, and music, Gloria speaks from a diverse menu of topics, ranging from health and business, to entertainment and spirituality.

Honored with the Lifetime Commitment Award from JDRF and the 1999 Woman of Achievement Award from the Miss America Organization, Loring is listed in the *World Who's Who of Women* and *Who's Who in America*. In her community, Gloria devotes her time and experience as President of the Lake Arrowhead Foundation for the Creative and Performing Arts. She is married to Emmy Award-winning art director and production designer, René Lagler. For more information, visit www.glorialoring.com.

DR. TIMOTHY J. GRAY, D.O., is board certified in Family Practice and is a Diabetic Educator. He's a Book-of-the-Month-Club author for both *Prevention* magazine and for Doubleday Book Club with *Backworks: The Illustrated Guide to How Your Back Works and What to Do When It Doesn't*.

Dr. Gray and his staff have participated in the Oregon Diabetes Collaborative. Several medical groups from Oregon working with OMPRO (Oregon Medical Peer Review Organization) have developed methods to measure excellence in diabetes care and programs to reach out to the community.

Dr. Gray has served on the Oregon Medical Association Medical Review Committee to help physicians update their practices and has served on the OMA PEER Group to help other physicians update their medical skills. He has also served as an Instructor in Human Anatomy at Pacific University and as an Assistant Clinical Instructor for the College of Osteopathic Medicine of the Pacific. He has been inducted into Sigma Sigma Phi, the National Osteopathic Fraternity for service to the profession.

As a diabetes educator, Dr. Gray knows that the deadliest fear in diabetes is that some patients have resigned themselves to, "My mother died of complications from diabetes and so will I," and hopes that by giving patients the tools to control their diabetes their condition won't have to control them.